LIFESMART
CAROLE CAPLIN

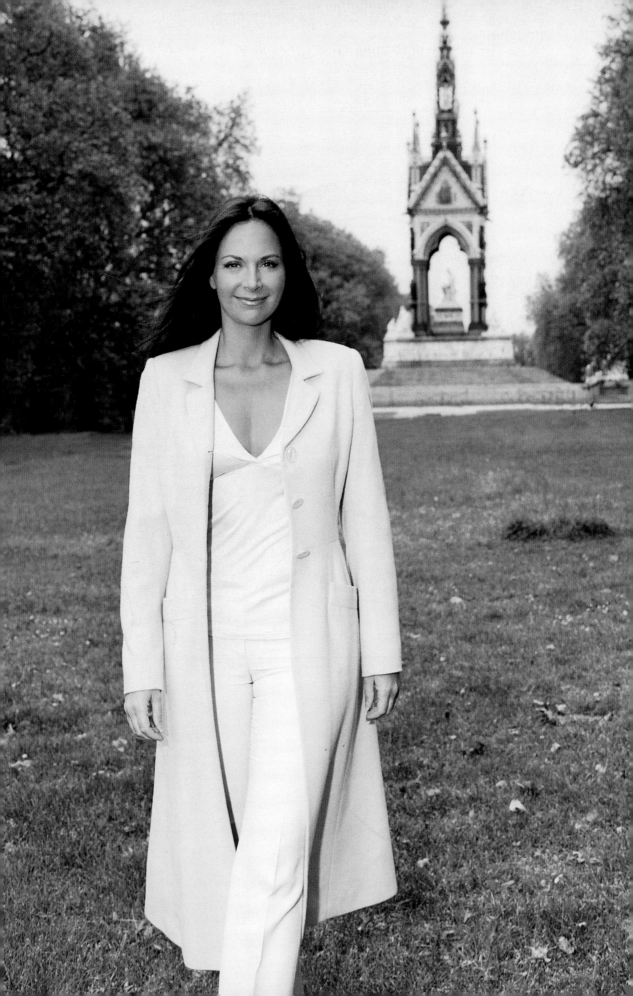

LIFESMART
CAROLE CAPLIN

GET THE FACTS, FOLLOW THE STEPS, FEEL THE DIFFERENCE

WEIDENFELD & NICOLSON

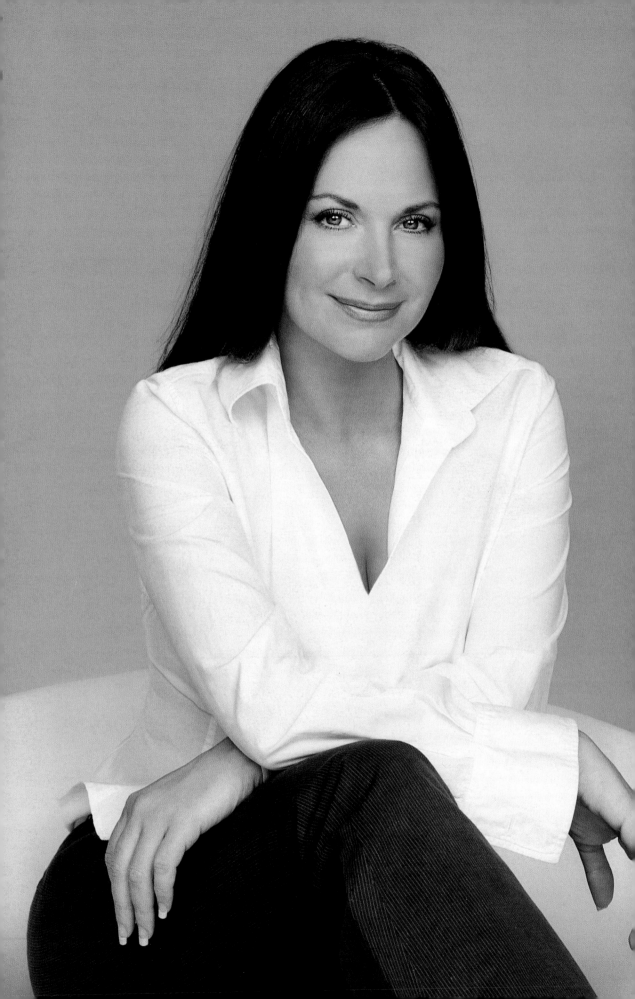

Contents

Carole on Her Soap Box

NOTHING MAKES ME HAPPIER than feeling really, really well.

This may sound like a rather simple thing to enjoy, but over the years I have come to realize that the feeling which comes from good health is a commodity worth far more than any precious stone. I've arrived at this point through a personal journey that has often involved walking into walls that I myself constructed. Being naturally stubborn and sceptical have proved to be both a curse and a blessing; both character traits have undoubtedly delayed – but then have helped – my own recovery. Don't get me wrong, I didn't have a life-threatening disease, but there was a period in my life when I suffered from a cocktail of modern-day maladies, including ME, candida, adult acne, severe scoliosis (curvature of the spine) and migraine. To add insult to injury, I also binge ate my way to being three stone over my normal weight. I was a 'high-flyer' working in sales and marketing when I reached my lowest point and was given some sharp home-truths about the state I was in. All this at the grand age of 22. Starting off on my journey, it took me many years to figure out the whys and wherefores of how to deal with my predicament.

No single person, belief system, therapy or advice was responsible for the outcome. It was the combination of a number of different resources and no-nonsense feedback, plus learning how to choose and manage those resources, that brought it all together for me. With this book, I would like to take you on a journey of investigation and discovery, so that you too can acquire the understanding and know-how necessary to be really well and happy. Rather than being prescriptive, my aim is to remove any prejudices, fears and preconceptions you may have, and to provide you with the information you need to make the choices that will benefit you.

In the early 1980s when I taught my first class, the worlds of complementary medicine and fitness were a far cry from today. Newspapers didn't report on health in nearly so much detail or in such a varied way as they do today. Since then, there have been thousands of health, fitness and lifestyle books, but the outstanding ones have been eclipsed by those advocating quick-fix, one-dimensional regimes that promise you instant results if you follow one person's magical advice.

Today, the health and fitness industries are larger and more powerful than ever, with gyms, spas and complementary health centres mushrooming. To keep up with this trend the media has massively increased its coverage of health-related issues in a mainly positive and proactive way. Health and lifestyle programmes seem to dominate television, and increasing numbers of complementary therapists, nutritionists and personal trainers are available countrywide. Yet over the same period, the incidence of sickness, obesity, cancer, depression and substance abuse has rocketed. It's as though we are in the grip of some sort of plague.

What is clear is that we need a broader, more thorough view of what it really will take to get us back on track. First though, I want to dispel any notion that this book is about

New Age mumbo-jumbo. I have derived immense benefit from exploring and incorporating the many activities that contribute to maintaining a healthy body, of which both orthodox and complementary approaches have a crucial role to play. Believing – or disbelieving – in any one philosophical approach is just not what LifeSmart is about. All I care about is what works; and to discover what works requires a genuinely open mind that is discerning and questioning, not arrogant and closed.

Anyone who jumps on any particular bandwagon is missing the point, and depriving themselves of alternative approaches that may potentially work for them. Partisan arguments about whether an approach is scientific or non-scientific are just a meaningless distraction. What *you* need to know is how to go about identifying – and then integrating in the right order – a mixture of whatever promotes optimum health and well-being for *you as an individual*, taking into account your own particular needs and problems.

Yet faced with so many medical and health practitioners working as one-dimensionally as they do, it's no wonder people constantly complain to me how hard it is to find out what's real, what works, and what doesn't. Particularly in the area of complementary medicine, I am often asked if I believe in something. My answer is always the same: I do not believe or disbelieve in anything. As far as I am concerned, it either works or it doesn't, and what works for one individual doesn't necessarily work for another...

Identifying for yourself your core issues and triggers, followed by what's available to you in every area and how to make use of it, will start you on your journey – and remember that the journey itself is just as important as the result. We have been so brainwashed about attaining instant results that we actually miss most of what we need to know if we are to achieve real, long-term change. Authors, practitioners and workers in all fields of health and fitness need to encourage the importance of the journey far more than the result itself.

CAROLE CAPLIN
LONDON

A Cynic's Tale

I FIRST WENT TO SEE CAROLE rather reluctantly. It was my girlfriend, now wife, Kay, who suggested it. And after I had ignored her suggestions for long enough, she pretty much insisted I went. Kay was a regular client of Carole's, primarily for general health, diet and keep fit purposes, but she had also been referred by Carole to Jack Temple, a complementary therapist. This put Carole firmly in the lunatic fringe as far I was concerned, even though Jack had successfully dealt with two considerable health issues that Kay had. I was quite certain that anything Carole did would not be founded upon anything remotely resembling sound medical principles.

In fact, 'sound medical principles' had not actually been doing me much good. My problem is simply that I have two distended discs in my lower back. I have been susceptible to back pain since childhood, but this had been exacerbated dramatically by a skiing accident about five years before. The basic symptom was that, with no particular warning, my back would periodically 'go', causing me acute pain, severely restricting mobility and, when the muscles then went into spasm, twisting my spine sideways such that I was unable to stand up straight. In extreme attacks, walking became virtually impossible and I was effectively confined to bed.

The problem had been gradually worsening ever since the skiing accident. Throughout this time I was receiving regular osteopathic and chiropractic care, some of which helped, some not. However, what became increasingly clear was that the treatment I was getting was at best alleviating the symptoms. It was certainly not solving the problem. By the end I was seeing a chiropractor three times a day. He would physically crunch my back into place so that I could walk out of his consulting room with my head held high, only to return a few hours later bent double.

Something had to be done. In my mind, however, this meant finding another chiropractor or osteopath who had a different approach. It most definitely did not mean anything at all unconventional. Indeed, it was only when I was advised that surgery was the sole option left that I panicked. Finally caving in to Kay's long-standing demands, I decided that trying something 'alternative' couldn't make it any worse and so I went to see Carole.

In that regard, Carole was something of a disappointment. She really didn't seem very alternative. At the time, she was not the public figure she has since become, so I didn't know what she looked like. In my mind, however, she was very definitely a tree-hugging earth mother who still worshipped planets or animal spirits. When I met her for the first time, however, she was practical, logical and full of common sense. With the minimum of preamble, she got me to lie on the floor and took me through a series of basic stretches and exercises. It was no miracle cure, but when I left 45 minutes later, the pain had eased a bit and there was clearly more mobility in my lower back. That was enough to persuade me to go back, and within a couple of months my back had improved beyond recognition.

I now see Carole once or twice a week at the gym for an hour of exercise. During this time I have come to realize that the reason she is so effective is that she cares a great deal about her clients, knows her stuff (which is unique to her style of teaching), has a good overview of all areas of health and has a strong and professional back-up team and network. The gym programme varies every visit, seemingly decided in line with how I and my back are feeling, but it is by no means exotic. It is generally made up of maintaining an open upper thorax while performing cardiovascular work; Carole's own remedial mobility and core stability exercises; conventional weight training; and a variety of breathing and stretching exercises.

To my surprise I have actually come to quite enjoy it. Carole is down-to-earth, speaks her mind and we usually have a laugh – at ourselves as much as anyone else. She has her foibles, such as some quite outrageous outfits or her determination to see if she can smell coffee on your breath when you're green with fatigue, but it is all done in good humour and she still smiles when you ignore her instructions completely. More important, however, is the end result. Other than through something self-induced such as lifting too heavy a weight in everyday life, my back is generally now absolutely fine and gives me no pain or restricted mobility at all. I see an osteopath in the same way I would visit my dentist, and the very real threat of surgery five years ago now seems a distant nightmare.

Acute back problems hamper a great deal of life's everyday activities. It is obvious that some things such as running, driving or carrying will be affected, but so too are countless other activities you normally don't even think about, such as getting up to answer the phone, leaning forward to clean your teeth or bending down to talk to a small child. For this reason, it is no exaggeration to say that Carole has transformed my quality of life. I have to say I never expected this to be the case when I originally and rather grudgingly agreed to go to see her. And even if I had, I would never have imagined in my wildest dreams that the 'weird and wacky' Carole Caplin would achieve it all simply through caring, common sense and a conventional exercise routine. If nothing else, I suppose that at least is a bit weird.

PAUL GOSWELL, Managing Director, property investment company

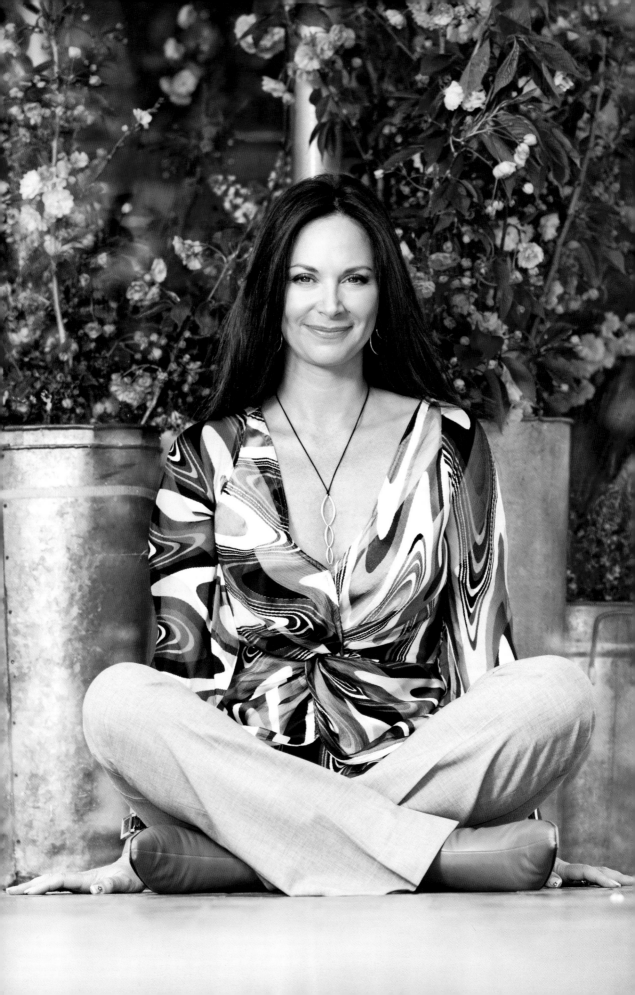

STARTERS
EXPAND YOUR IDEAS

So What's Going Wrong?

MOST PEOPLE THESE DAYS constantly feel below par, as if their bodies have gone way out of control. And not only do they not know where to start to remedy the problem, often they don't even have the inclination to do so. Too many people are uncomfortable with their bodies but aren't prepared to take any exercise. Even those who are motivated may eat the most perfect diet but find they are still not losing weight; or they exercise regularly, but still do not attain the shape they desire.

We are more disconnected from our bodies than we have ever been. It's as if over the last 50 years there's been a slow dumbing down of our own systems and how we look after ourselves. Any quick fix, from fast food to antibiotics, has taken over. Throughout the same period, there's been a huge shift in the roles men and women play. Women are constantly being challenged to allow both their femininity and career goals to exist side by side. Men are struggling to adapt to the changing roles of women, while still being expected to be the 'archetypal man'. Children and teenagers are facing more challenges and pressures than ever before. The problem is, we haven't taken the time to assimilate the myriad changes these profound social shifts have brought about.

Meanwhile, the competition for the money in our pockets has coloured and tainted everything available to us pharmaceutically and medically. We are bombarded with countless advertising and media images, which endlessly churn reams of information in and out of our lives. This encourages pointless envy and greed and saps energy. It also prevents us from getting the simple, basic information we need for physical and emotional health and well-being.

External Influences

Have we as a society become more destructively self-obsessed? I believe so. Never before have so many of our absolute needs been met so absolutely. Most of us enjoy a high material standard of living and a relatively easy, comfortable life; yet as a society we are getting more and more depressed. It's as if the more we have, the more we expect as a right. We are obsessed with comparing ourselves to other people, and have never been so flooded by messages about how we should look, dress, act and behave, what we should own and the work we should do.

There is a huge emphasis on the aesthetic, 'the look', and whether something's fashionable or sexy, yet not on basic good health and well-being. On an emotional level, our society seems more fragmented and splintered than ever before. Far too many people try to deal with their emotional problems by taking drugs, prescription or otherwise, and drug-taking is now at epidemic levels.

'Getting out of your head' used to be associated with youth experimentation and rebellion, but not any more. Today, in many quarters, you're virtually a social outcast if you do not partake of the drug of the evening. Respected professional people of all ages, married couples with children, city and country dwellers and celebrities have fallen prey in their droves – to recreational drugs, cocaine and cannabis in particular. Whatever the cause, this is a problem that is affecting every aspect of modern-day life and behaviour.

What You Think:	What Actually Happens:
Helps you to fit in and bond	You just feel isolated when you come out the other end.
Makes you happy	Emphasizes how sad you really are, and drugs act as a depressant when the initial effects have worn off.
Gives you a buzz and a high	You have a massive low to look forward to.
Increases energy	You have to keep taking more and more to reach the same peak, leaving every part of you exhausted.
Gets rid of your inhibitions	It increases your paranoia, awkwardness and self-consciousness.
Gives you an excuse to do stupid things	Drugs separate you from any form of intimacy. It numbs your feelings – both good and bad. It deepens your insecurity and kills any emotional intelligence and know-how. Finally, it disconnects you from others and if you don't stop, you end up dead.
Makes you forget your problems	It exacerbates your problems – they just get bigger. What you resist persists.
Makes you believe you are cool	Get real. I can't begin to tell you that, no matter how gorgeous, intelligent, moneyed, gifted and tragic you are, you have no idea just how uncool and unsexy drugs actually are.
It will get you attention	At what cost?

If people aren't taking illegal drugs, then alcohol is just around the corner. And if that isn't enough, the constant drip-feed of painkillers, antibiotics, steroids and any other medication should really put the boot in. Poor diet is just the icing on the cake.

Lack Of Integration

Nowadays, we have more choice of alternative solutions to medical problems than ever before. Yet there are still many individuals who either don't know anything about complementary medicine or wouldn't dare to explore what it has to offer. Those who do go to see complementary practitioners, receiving immediate and often remarkable benefits, often sabotage the results by not following up the practitioner's long-term recommendations.

At the moment, too many orthodox medical practitioners, complementary therapists and other health and fitness experts work independently of each other, not as an integrated team. What's more, many people either don't understand the necessity of incorporating good nutrition and exercise to back up their external therapies, or they can't be bothered to. Instead of utilizing these health-care resources in a preventative or transformative way, they merely plaster over the cracks.

We need to understand that everything affecting our bodies is intrinsically linked – the stresses we're subjected to, the junk food we ingest and the products we use – and we shouldn't compartmentalize what we do to be healthy. For example, often we go on a diet, join a gym or see a complementary practitioner in total isolation from everything else we're doing. Results either do not occur at all, or drop away after an initial surge because we are not looking at the whole picture. I'm not talking about needing to be a fitness fanatic or a health freak, but about you having all the information that you need in order to make the right choices so that good health becomes second nature. This is what your school didn't teach you and your parents probably didn't know.

If schools taught proper nutritional education – and emulated that in the food they dish up – and we had been taught how to breathe and stand correctly, isolate and coordinate, along with other physical and emotional knowledge, this book would not be necessary. If we were warned about the dangers of toxic chemicals and junk food, and knew how to use orthodox and complementary approaches appropriately, I would happily have very little work to do.

Think of health and well-being as being like a giant, interconnected jigsaw puzzle. Any area to do with your day-to-day life and personality is a part of the puzzle that has to be incorporated in order to achieve sustainable results. If you target different areas simultaneously, rather than just one in isolation, the puzzle will eventually be solved.

Self-infliction

Wouldn't it be great to start each day feeling like you do when you've had a week's holiday? I don't mean a boozing, up all night, out in the sun all day frying type of

• A Mori study in 2003 found that one in five Britons suffer from stress every day; the most common causes of stress being jobs and money.

holiday. But a real sleeping, daydreaming, collapse, relax and let it all go break. After several days on this kind of holiday you wake up with a physical sensation in your bones, muscles, skin and eyes of feeling really, really well. Sounds great, doesn't it? So why are we are not allowing this to be the case every day?

Life In The Fast Lane

These days we have so little time to digest any area of our lives that we find ourselves consistently running behind, often having to sacrifice time with children, family and partners to stay ahead of the game.

The thought of slowing down or missing out on anything seems like a threat. That's life in the fast lane – not much time for anything of real value at all.

Energy Levels

Whether it is self-inflicted or not, both adults and children are constantly pushed and under pressure to perform and produce, plus we don't get the hours of sleep we need at the right times. As a result of this, our systems are worn down through constant fatigue. To add insult to injury, when we do get ill we don't recuperate in the way we should. We either keep going through will-power, or we put our bodies through multiple physical workouts combined with an over-abundance of supplements, being extremely proud of the way we never have a day off work because of illness. Either way, these approaches are likely to leave us prone to constant minor illnesses. Allowing one's immune system to crash when it's had enough is more productive in the long run, because overriding your system constantly will just get you into deeper trouble.

When we lose touch with our bodies, we don't know how to read them and we don't trust our own healing process. Ted Mortar, who pioneered the therapy technique BEST (see page 42) communicates the idea eloquently. 'Those who say a particular health therapy can cure everything are inaccurate. All curing and healing is done by the body – period. All therapies do is aid nature in her quest for normality to restore and maintain health. Nature is not only smarter than we think; nature is smarter than we *can* think.'

Stuck In A Rut

We tend to stick to the environment we work, travel and live in, and not enough of us get a change of scenery. We no longer adjust to the seasons with our food or our activities – it's all too easy to stay indoors in the darker months – and we don't plan enough in advance to break out of our workaday lives with recreational and relaxing pursuits.

The time that we waste – for instance, arguing with our partners for reasons we can't even remember, or putting everyone else first – stops us from creating the necessary personal space we need to deal with everything that affects us. We socialize endlessly because of the fear that we will be missing out, often leaving ourselves exhausted and run down, and we eat and drink when often we actually don't really enjoy or need it. Breaking this cycle and going out only when we really want to may seem impossible, but doing so allows us enough time to recoup in order for us to service our busy lives and to maintain our energy levels, our sense of perspective and our good health.

Medicating Your Detox

It has recently become ultra-fashionable to detox from binge living every now and again. However, most people usually medicate their detoxification process within a few hours of starting it – in other words replacing one form of toxin with another. For example, as the headache is just about to hit, they take a painkiller; having given up smoking, people suck on sweets or gorge on food instead.

The fact is that when you give up cigarettes, alcohol, or certain addictive food stuffs, such as caffeine and chocolate, it's not only your physical body that's detoxifying. It's your emotional body too. Subconsciously our systems want to fill the gap and we can do that by overdoing work or sport and by filling every spare minute of the day. Learning to understand what's fully involved in giving something up, and what the physical, emotional and psychological reactions and repercussions can be, is therefore vital.

Fear Of Change

The thought of personal change can be very threatening. The mind tends to perceive that any change, even for the better, is unsafe and not worth the risk. Some people argue that change is unnecessary or a waste of time. Whatever threat an individual registers, any suggestion of change almost always elicits cynicism, aggression, lies or bullying. Whatever the reaction, it is usually just an excuse to avoid change.

Yet life is all about change. There is a constant process in our bodies of shedding, replacement and renewal. For optimum health, we need to do everything necessary to ensure those processes can go on unimpaired.

Change requires openness and cooperation, and timing is vital. If there's one thing I have learnt over the years, it's that nobody can be forced to change, and it's no use trying. All you can do is appeal to someone's best instincts, make suggestions, then leave it at that. Destructive relationships occur when a long-suffering partner tries every possible way to get the other person to change, failing to realize that the only person they have the power to change and move forward is, of course, themselves. Fear of change happens when we get stuck in our ways, greedy or desperate to keep our status, earning capacity and power.

Stereotypes

Although we have access to all sorts of excellent information these days, the media often still tries to fit issues about health into outdated stereotypes. So, medicine is written about as an either/or option between orthodox and complementary. Depending on the publication's agenda, an article may appear negatively in the investigative part of the paper one day and positively in the health part several weeks or months later.

Yet the truth about stereotyping today is that it has largely disappeared. Most of us refuse to fit into narrow little boxes any more. We like mix and we like variety. We are enjoying expressing the different sides of our personality in our choice of music, cuisine and fashion. People are prepared to cross boundaries in order to have a mix of experiences in all areas, whether culture, religion, sport or travel. So it really is rather strange that when it comes to alternative and complementary health, parts of the media still feel the need to attack solutions which don't conform to outmoded preconceptions!

An Integrated Approach

One of the single most exciting aspects of researching and writing this book has been discovering how many professionals in the orthodox medical sphere – doctors, dentists, nurses and therapists – are now seriously seeking to integrate their work with preventative, holistic, complementary medical approaches.

I believe this is because more and more people are recognizing that as a society, we simply do not have the time or resources to deal with the ever-increasing numbers of ill people simply by diagnosing existing symptoms and then suggesting drugs or surgery. We need to look at more preventative and complementary measures as we have a huge overload of sickness already, and an NHS groaning under the strain.

It is far too easy for conservative people, with their own vested interests in maintaining the status quo, to damn more innovative practitioners, whose work and theories they barely understand, let alone want to. My advice is: if you have a health problem, whether conventional medicine has the answers or not, check out alternative approaches for yourself. All that matters is what works best for you.

You may well be put off by a number of factors when exploring complementary practices. Negative feedback includes the unappealing personal appearance of some practitioners, their use of irritating jargon, an abrupt bedside manner or being over-emphatic in their views. However, the same can be said for orthodox practitioners. The trick is to get whatever value you can from any of these individuals and discard what doesn't benefit you.

Only a few of the problems with our health and well-being are insurmountable. With sufficient knowledge and awareness, we have the power in our own hands to choose a combination of what works for us in order to tackle what's going wrong. Once you have the know-how and the tools, when you understand it all takes time and there's no quick fix, and you've come to know yourself a little better, you'll be able to negotiate between your levels of self-sabotage and will-power. All I'm asking you to do is to take a whole body approach, which means looking at everything including stress factors, your environment, and your physical and emotional health. No matter what your current state of well-being, your life in this day and age could be better. Much better.

• In the four years since 1999–2000, the number of prescriptions issued in the UK has increased by 22 per cent to 632 million in total, costing the NHS almost 50 per cent more than it did four years ago.

Choices And Consequences – Issues In Today's World

We all want to be healthy and have a good quality of life. So why is it that so many of the choices we make, either personally or as a community, lead directly to ill health and a very poor quality of life?

One of the main problems is that we naturally want to trust and do so en masse without bothering to question. We trust in science and technology, in the expertise of medical specialists and pharmaceutical companies, and in the vigilance of government experts to safeguard the quality of our food and water, the products we buy and the services we use. These choices affect our beliefs and attitudes and are virtually forced upon us by big multinational corporations who are driven by financial considerations, or sometimes even by governments and public health authorities. But maybe we shouldn't be so complacent. The trouble is, it is human nature to accept the status quo, trusting that 'the authorities' know best, and that they would never knowingly condone anything that could harm public health. We assume, for instance, that products on sale in our supermarkets must be safe. Otherwise they'd be banned, wouldn't they?

Let me give you an example. A couple of decades ago we were all strongly urged not to eat butter because it was a saturated fat and was therefore bad for us. Many food companies jumped on this bandwagon and started manufacturing and marketing margarine instead, which was made from hydrogenated fat. Various public health agencies backed this 100 per cent – only to realize years later that the trans fatty acids in hydrogenated fat are implicated in coronary disease. Now there's a campaign in the US – where it all started – to remove trans fats from all cakes, snacks and fast foods. In 2002, a US expert committee on nutrition concluded that there was no level of trans fat in the diet that could be deemed safe. Now, we're being told to eat butter again.

Not questioning what's going on around us appears to save time, energy and money. But we pay a heavy price. The vast majority of us have no idea of the toxic chemicals in our food, make-up or shaving lotions, our daily skincare and bath products, household products, medicines and drugs, or even the clothes we wear.

Most people also have no idea how exposure to these chemicals can sabotage their efforts to have an efficient immune system, and in many cases is the mystery factor responsible for unsuccessful attempts to lose weight or fight off recurring minor illnesses. Most people also seem totally unaware of how the chemically treated, repeatedly recycled tap water they drink and bathe in is saturating their bodies in chlorine and female hormones, or of the carcinogens and other toxic substances in hundreds of popular household cleaning products, cosmetics and shampoos that cause myriad health-related problems.

There is increasing awareness of the dangers of over-prescribing antibiotics and antidepressants, of adding fluoride and chlorine to water supplies, and of spraying foodstuffs with herbicides and pesticides. Mass consumer protest is holding off the introduction of genetically modified (GM) crops and food throughout Europe. Increasingly, ordinary people are even beginning to question the wisdom of modern-day immunisation schedules for tiny babies and toddlers, which is still one of orthodox medicine's most sacred cows.

Yet too many people are still burying their heads in the sand, either refusing to take responsibility or thinking that somehow none of the warnings and worrying statistics applies to them. The quick-fix, instant gratification, least-output-for-the-fastest-result approach remains the biggest selling point. If there's one thing that most people are focused on, it's the short term.

I've lost count of the number of people I've seen who smoke, drink a lot of coffee and/or alcohol, take antibiotics for recurring illnesses, don't drink water and surround themselves with chemically based products – and who cannot understand why they feel exhausted, depressed and no matter how hard they try, cannot lose weight or get well.

My view is simple. If you're interested in keeping yourself and your children as healthy and well as possible, then you need to invest time and energy and, where necessary, money, to minimize your exposure to chemicals and all other artificial, man-made products and substances. I believe in keeping things as natural as possible: eating organic biodynamic produce that is fresh and unprocessed; wearing clothes that are made out of natural fibres where possible; choosing glass over plastic containers when you can; and using biodegradable, plant-based products in every area of daily living. That way, when we do use or ingest anything that is synthetic or toxic, our bodies are far better able to deal with the repercussions. Unwanted consequences can never be completely avoided, but the way to minimize them is to make choices that are as well-informed as possible. You need to be aware of how the environment all around you, and what is being done to it, affects every aspect of your health, well-being and state of mind.

The following are some of the most significant health and environmental issues facing all of us living in highly industrialized Western societies today.

Immunisation

On one side of the immunisation debate is the entire orthodox medical establishment, urging parents to vaccinate their babies and young children without hesitation, and warning of dire health consequences if they do not. On the other side, there are many committed opponents who believe the procedure compromises babies' and very young children's developing auto-immune system and does more harm than good, including being a major contributing factor to the explosive rise in the number of children with autism, bowel problems and other complaints.

The dilemma for parents is that they are being asked to weigh up all sorts of statistically small but extremely worrying risks, with many suspecting that they are not being given all the information available. Will my child be left with autism, brain damage or some other form of disability if I follow the urgings of doctors and the health authorities and vaccinate? But if I don't vaccinate, what are the chances

• The number of children diagnosed with autism has rocketed from one in 2,500 ten years ago to one in 166 today. There's no official explanation as to why. Autism is now more common than multiple sclerosis, cystic fibrosis or childhood cancer.

that my child may get gravely ill or even die from measles, mumps or some other childhood illness?

Then there is the question of each person's responsibility to the wider community. If I reject immunisation, my child may be fine, but what if he or she passes on rubella to a pregnant woman, or infects other children with a contagious disease, as doctors warn?

In the end, we must all decide for ourselves, but my personal view is that immunisation is not the panacea it is so often presented as being, but a medicalised form of Russian roulette. If I were a parent, I would think very deeply about the pros and cons of each type of vaccination. I think it is perfectly reasonable for parents to ask doctors: what is the actual risk of my child catching a particular disease – tetanus at three months of age, for instance – compared to the impact of multi-vaccines on a very fragile and developing immune system, brain and nervous system? Although mercury has now been taken out of children's vaccines, an impressive bunch of undesirable ingredients still remain. These have the potential to produce adverse reactions, and are also present in adult vaccines.

For more information, visit www.mercola.com and What Doctors Don't Tell You at www.wddty.co.uk.

A much fuller account of the immunisation debate can be found at www.lifesmart.co.uk, but for the official view on why all children should be immunised, visit the Department of Health website, www.dh.gov.uk.

For more information on the risks associated with childhood immunisations and research references, visit www.informedparent.co.uk, or call The Informed Parent helpline on 01903 212 969.

Water Quality

Nothing is more essential to good health than an adequate daily intake of clean, pure water. Every day, the body loses up to two-and-a-half litres of fluid through the skin, lungs, guts and kidneys, and that water needs to be replaced. That's why, depending on size, physical output and environmental conditions, we need to drink between one-and-a-half and two-and-a-half litres of water a day.

But what sort of water should we drink? In the UK, the government body responsible for safeguarding the quality of public water supplies, the Drinking Water Inspectorate (DWI), asserts that our tap water is of an extremely high quality and is entirely safe to drink. Tap water is not only just as good as the bottled variety, the DWI says, but often a good deal fresher, since bottles can sit in warehouses and on supermarket shelves for up to two years.

However, bottled water is now a billion-pound-a-year industry in Britain, and millions of us buy it assuming it's purer and healthier than tap water, which can legally be contaminated by bacteria, herbicides, pesticides, lead, nitrates from fertilizers, aluminium residues and chlorine, which is added as a disinfectant. (One problem with chlorine in tap water is that it enters the body through the skin and lungs every time we take a shower or bath. A 15-minute hot shower exposes the body to more by-products of this gas than drinking eight glasses of water.)

Yet some bottled waters have such high sodium levels that they can be a risk to people with high blood pressure or heart disease. Fluoride levels can also be relatively high in bottled water, although in Britain it's not compulsory to state the fluoride content. Even calcium levels are too high in many bottled brands, particularly if there's not enough magnesium present to enable the calcium to be absorbed properly, leading to calcification in soft tissues and arteries. This, in turn, can adversely affect bone density – the very opposite of what we assume calcium's effects to be.

All this makes it essential to check the fine print on the labels of bottled water, and only to buy those brands with very low sodium, low calcium and high magnesium levels. Also, always check how long there is to go before the use-by date, so that you buy water that is as fresh as possible.

Finally, there's the choice between plastic and glass bottles. Glass is preferable, as plastic can leach chemicals and bacteria into the water, particularly if left in the sun for any length of time, or if all the water is not drunk immediately once opened. See www.lifesmart.co.uk for more information and alternative recommendations.

The Drinking Water Inspectorate is at www.dwi.gov.uk, or call 0207 082 8024. The water industry also supplies information at www.water.org.uk.

For information on bottled water, visit the International Bottled Water Association at www.bottledwater.org, or the US Environmental News Network website at www.enn.com.

Fluoridation

Fluoridation sounds great – in theory at least. Add some fluoride to public water supplies and rates of tooth decay among children decline dramatically. Decades of toothpaste advertising have also left us with an image of fluoride as a cute, cuddly sort of chemical additive. Unfortunately, this is far from the case. In anything but the most minute quantities, fluoride is a highly poisonous substance. The side effects of over-exposure range from dental fluorosis – meaning mottled enamel – to musculoskeletal, immune system, metabolic and central nervous system damage.

Of particular concern to many scientists is the accumulating evidence that fluoride attacks the thyroid system, resulting in chronic ill health, fatigue, atherosclerosis and heart attacks, depression and obesity. It does this by displacing iodine, essential for the manufacture of thyroid hormone. At the same time, natural iodine levels in our foodstuffs are falling steadily. If we are not getting enough iodine in our daily diets, that is a matter for grave public concern. Iodine deficiency in pregnant women, for example, can result in major damage to unborn babies, in particular affecting their central nervous system.

As evidence of the damage of over-exposure to fluoride has accumulated, fluoridation has been discontinued in many countries. Now, except for a small area in northern Spain, southern Ireland and around 10 per cent of the UK, fluoridation has been banned throughout Europe, as well as in Japan and China. Basel in Switzerland was one of the last European authorities to act, stopping the practice in 2003 after a scientific review. In 2002, Belgium also banned the sale of fluoride tablets, drops and chewing gum.

Yet amazingly, the British government is swimming against this international tide of scientific opinion and public concern, passing legislation in late 2003 to give local health authorities the power to order water suppliers to add fluoride.

Tooth decay is not caused by lack of fluoride but by too much highly refined, sugary food and drink, and by people not cleaning their teeth properly. I believe that the answer to tooth decay is not to force a registered poison with no medicinal authorization on the entire population, many of whom have specifically withheld their consent, but to educate people, particularly parents of young children, about the real causes of tooth decay.

If you live in an area where fluoride has already been added to the public water supply, or is to be added, the case for installing a household water purification system becomes far stronger. You can also use an alternative natural fluoride toothpaste (see page 207).

For more information, visit www.npwa.freeserve.co.uk or call 01226 360 909.

'Frankenfoods' – The GM Monster

Genetic modification is an unproven food technology that plucks a gene from one living being, animal or plant, and inserts it into the genetic make-up of another, thus 'modifying' it. No one knows what the long-term effects will be. Worldwide, there have been only 10 published studies looking at the effect of genetically modified (GM) foods on the human body. Five of these studies, which were connected to the biotechnology companies involved in developing and selling GM seeds, found no harmful effects. The other five independent studies identified worrying changes in the human gut which have yet to be explained or studied further. Farmers are also now reporting unusual effects in animals eating GM feed, including birth defects; although, again, these are rarely investigated or followed up.

Why, you might well ask, would anyone in their right mind be arguing that GM crops be planted, until – and unless – we know with absolute certainty that GM foods are safe? The answer is a depressingly familiar one. The push for GM comes from giant American agrochemical companies, chief among them Monsanto.

Anything occurring naturally cannot be patented. Once any organism is modified in a laboratory, however, it can be patented and then marketed. And that, in the end, explains the development of GM seeds.

In the US and Canada, where GM crops are now widespread, hundreds of farmers are now being sued on the basis that they used a genetically modified seed without license. Yet the seeds may well have turned up by accident, as seeds do, transported by bees or the wind. Indeed, this potential for contamination is one of the major reasons campaigners have long argued against GM crops in the first place.

Genetic engineers claim this technology is in their control, and is controllable. But I believe that nothing could be further from reality. Inserting a gene where it does not belong randomly disrupts its new neighbouring genes. In addition, in order to insert a gene, it is packaged inside a bacterium so it will successfully invade an organism. Unlike traditional breeding practices, genetic engineering is based on the same invasive forces as an infectious disease.

Biologist and Nobel Laureate in Medicine George Wald says that genetic engineering 'places in human hands the capacity to redesign living organisms, the products of some three billion years of evolution. Such intervention must not be confused with previous intrusions upon the natural order of living organisms; animal and plant breeding, for example. All such earlier procedures worked within single or closely related species. The nub of the new technology is to move genes back and forth, not only across species lines, but across any boundaries that now divide living organisms.'

Despite intense pressure from the US, including the outrageous threat of trade sanctions, Europe has so far managed to keep GM foodstuffs at bay. In Britain, every opinion poll on the issue has consistently shown that most people do not want anything to do with GM foods. Yet in early 2004, the Government gave the go-ahead for a variety of GM maize to be grown as animal feed.

It is crystal clear that one thing, and one thing alone, will keep GM crops out of Britain. And that is consumer pressure.

Supporters of GM crops reportedly think public opposition will eventually be 'worn down'. I beg to differ. If anything, the public's rejection of GM is just getting stronger and stronger. As a result, companies developing GM crops have been avoided by investors and research funding is now drying up.

The British government's Science Review Panel, established to advise on whether GM crops are safe or not, admits that GM and organic agriculture cannot coexist because contamination is inevitable, and that a choice will have to be made between the two. Good. Forced to choose, I think we can predict with absolute confidence what anyone in their right mind would decide. Let's all just hope and pray that it is people in their right mind who have the final say.

For information on how to join the international campaign against GM foods, visit Friends of the Earth at www.foe.co.uk, GeneWatch UK at www.genewatch.org, or Greenpeace at www.greenpeace.org.uk.

Global Warming And What You Can Do

It is easy to assume that there's not a lot that any of us as individuals can do about reversing climate change, which perhaps explains why so many of us are in denial about the fact that it is already underway. Research conducted by the UK Energy Saving Trust (EST) in August 2003 revealed that 85 per cent of Britons believe that the effects of climate change will not be seen for decades, while seven per cent think it will never happen.

EST Chief Executive Philip Sellwood believes these views are sadly deluded. Climate change, he says, is a reality. In 2003 alone, the UK experienced an unprecedented combination of record temperatures, tornadoes and flooding. 'Despite these clear signs, most people are still not acknowledging the effect their actions are having on the environment,' Sellwood says.

In the UK, one-quarter of all carbon dioxide emissions – one of the leading contributors to climate change – comes from energy use at home. According to the EST, much of this energy – an estimated £96 million worth every week – could be saved. 'Being energy efficient in the home is common sense and easy – everyone can do it, every day, whether it be turning off the light when leaving the room or insulating your cavity walls,' Sellwood says. 'The average household can save up to £200 a year by taking up energy efficiency measures, a saving of around two tonnes of carbon dioxide emission.'

The Energy Saving Trust, which was established by the UK Government after the 1992 Earth Summit in Rio de Janeiro, is one of the UK's leading organizations addressing the damaging effects of climate change. A non-profit organization, the EST aims to cut carbon dioxide emissions by promoting the sustainable and efficient use of energy, offering UK households free, expert and impartial advice on how to become more energy efficient.

For more information, visit www.saveenergy.co.uk or call 0845 727 7200.

Organic Farming And Food

The rise of the organic food movement is one of the best, most heartening developments of recent decades. If you care about your family's health, the environment and animal welfare, one of the single most effective things you can do as a consumer is support organic and biodynamic farming methods.

Organic farmers reject the chemical fertilizers, pesticides and herbicides that have so depleted the soil, damaged wildlife and poisoned our food. All artificial flavours and colours are banned from organic produce, and many dubious additives have never been allowed in organic food, including phosphoric acid, aspartame, hydrogenated fat and monosodium glutamate.

Organic standards have also, since the 1990s, banned any foodstuffs containing GM ingredients, including animal feed. The very existence of organic agriculture has been one of the main arguments against the introduction of GM crops because of the risk of wind- or insect-borne contamination.

Chemical fertilizers are, without doubt, a quick way to feed a crop. Instead of time-consuming composting – where waste organic matter rots down into crumbly, nutrient-rich earth – chemical nutrients are added. But over time, this method takes more out of the soil than it puts back in, resulting in a depleted soil with fewer nutrients on offer. Figures from the UK Department of Agriculture show that, between 1940 and 1991, mineral levels in UK fruit and vegetables have fallen catastrophically, some by as much as 76 per cent.

Then there's the use of herbicides and pesticides; can residues enter – and accumulate in – our bodies? In 2004, the World Wide Fund for Nature took blood samples from 47 people, and found, on average, 41 chemical compounds in their blood. One chemical detected was DDT, even though this pesticide has been banned since the 1970s because of its potential to cause cancer as well as its devastating impact on wildlife.

It is notoriously hard to scientifically prove the health benefits of eating organic food – but surely it is common sense to avoid food laced with toxic chemicals?

Organic food is not just about keeping toxic chemicals out but also about taking more health-giving nutrients in. Research shows that eating organic food significantly increases your intake of beneficial vitamins, minerals, essential fats and antioxidants.

Organic farming also aims to farm with the least ecological damage possible, and as its standards require respect for animals' natural behaviour and diet it benefits farm animals. There has been not one incidence of BSE in cattle born and reared on an organic farm in Britain.

Non-organic food is widely bought, mainly because it is almost always cheaper than organic food, particularly in supermarkets. There are a number of reasons for the difference in costs, including the fact that organic crops are grown on a smaller scale and non-organic food is actually subsidised by the taxpayers.

What price can you put on health? Surely it is more precious than, say, a pair of trainers? I strongly believe that the extra money spent on organic food is worth it. You are not only buying into a farming system that is kinder to wildlife and the environment, but you are also getting in return a quality product that is keeping toxic chemicals out of your body, boosting your vitality and protecting your health.

The Soil Association suggests ways to save money when buying organic food. First, buy fresh seasonal organic produce direct from the farmer, either from a farmers' market, farm shop or using a box delivery scheme. This is often cheaper than buying the same produce at a supermarket, and as it is locally grown, it is also far fresher than produce that has travelled vast distances, so it tastes better too.

Organic meat costs more because of the higher standards of animal welfare. But you can keep costs down by cooking with less meat – try bulking up a casserole with lentils or extra vegetables. Alternatively, save your organic roast for a special occasion like Sunday lunch.

The UK Soil Association has a network of organic farms that are open to the public. Log on to www.soilassociation.org or call 0117 314 5000.

The Association also sells an Organic Directory that gives up-to-date listings of organic box schemes, local farmers' markets and shops.

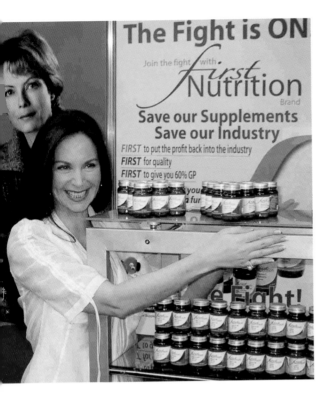

Jenny Seagrove and
Carole at the Natural
Health Show 2004 on
the First Nutrition stand
fighting the cause to
save our supplements.

The EU Threat To Consumer Choice

In a world awash with legally available substances that maim, kill and cause havoc — cigarettes, alcohol and junk food being the most obvious examples — the last thing you might expect governments to be considering banning would be vitamin and mineral supplements and traditional herbal remedies. Think again. Unbelievably, a raft of EU legislation now threatens consumer access to a huge range of these natural health care products.

Under a European Commission directive, which the British Government has accepted without demur, an estimated 5,000 vitamin and mineral formulations will become illegal from August 2005 and will disappear from our shops. Any shopkeeper who does continue to sell them — as many propose defiantly to do — will be committing a criminal offence.

Only vitamins and minerals that are on an approved 'Positive List' can be sold legally — and at the moment, this List excludes 250 nutrients which British consumers have been using safely for decades. Manufacturers can submit dossiers of detailed scientific data to support applications for inclusion on the List, but producing these dossiers is incredibly expensive and many manufacturers will be unable to afford it. As a result, British consumers will be denied access to hundreds of safe nutrients — minerals such as boron and selenium, and numerous forms of vitamins A, C and E — many of which have been on sale for years without problem.

From October 2005, under another EU Directive, herbal products can only be sold if they have been in traditional medicinal use for at least 30 years and are produced to expensive standards more appropriate to pharmaceutical drugs. Again, cost pressures will force many smaller manufacturers out of business.

Millions of people who wish to use supplements and herbal remedies will have their freedom of choice drastically curtailed, a thriving industry will be all but wiped out, and thousands of people will lose their jobs. So while off-licences and fast-food outlets can continue to peddle anything they want, however demonstrably injurious to health, the small health food shop next door will be all but driven out of business.

Amazingly, of course, this comes at a time when studies are increasingly showing that modern farming methods and plant-breeding techniques, as already discussed, are stripping basic foodstuffs of many of the vitamins and minerals essential for human health. Over the past 60 years, the levels of iron, magnesium, potassium, copper and other minerals essential for the body's biochemical balance have dropped in fruit and vegetables by up to three-quarters. In addition, low levels of trace elements in the diet have been linked to obesity, insulin resistance, heart disease and mental illness. Yet in future, many of the food supplements that millions of us buy to boost our intake of trace elements and vitamins will be banned.

The EU argues that these measures are essential 'to protect consumers' – yet no evidence has ever been produced to show that any of the products due to be banned are unsafe.

Britain, Holland and Ireland have always had a far more liberal approach to vitamins and mineral supplements than other European countries, but to enforce uniformity, the EU decided that Britain, Holland and Ireland should be brought in line with the rest of the EU. And as far as reasons go, that's about it.

For more information, visit Consumers For Health Choice at www.healthchoice.org,uk, or ask for advice at your local health food store.

Quitting Smoking And The NRT Scandal

If you're a smoker thinking of trying to quit, you will almost certainly find yourself directed towards Nicotine Replacement Therapy, or NRT – patches, gum, lozenges and the like, made by pharmaceutical companies. Over the past decade or so, NRT has been enthusiastically adopted by all the official quit smoking authorities around the world as the only method 'proven' to help smokers stop. In Britain, it's now available on NHS prescription, as well as over-the-counter in pharmacies and supermarkets. The problem is, NRT doesn't actually work very well.

Although clinical trials indicate that NRT doubles a smoker's chances of quitting and not smoking for over 12 months, it only doubles it from around three per cent, using will-power alone, to six per cent. Smokers attending NHS clinics have about a 10 per cent chance of quitting using will-power alone, compared with 20 per cent using NRT.

• Each year, 120,000 people in the UK die from smoking and a further 12,000 die from passive smoking.

That may sound quite impressive, until you realize that the best quit smoking methods around the world achieve a success rate well in excess of 50 per cent. What are these methods? They are educationally based rather than medically based methods that explain convincingly to smokers *not why they shouldn't smoke* – since everyone knows that by now – *but why they do smoke*.

When you think about it, that indeed is the key question. Smokers know that they are ingesting poisonous substances which will almost certainly damage their health sooner or later, and are paying through the nose to do so. The average 20-a-day smoker spends £1,700 a year on cigarettes, and prices are going up all the time. Why on earth would anyone spend all that money to risk a slow and agonizing death from some awful smoking-related disease?

Smokers smoke because they are addicted to nicotine and, like any addicts, are experts at rationalizing away the grave harm they are doing to both their health

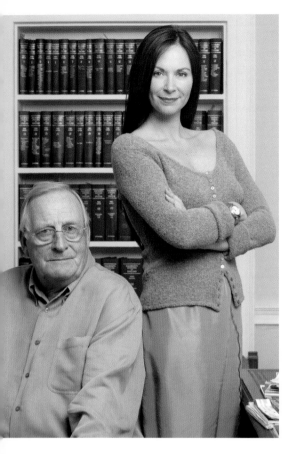

Allen Carr and Carole together to back Allen's way of helping people to give up smoking the natural way.

and pockets. The best quit smoking methods are the ones that help smokers to see through the illusions which fuel their addiction – the belief, for instance, that nicotine helps to calm the nerves when actually it just makes smokers edgier – and help them to understand that they can cope with life's stresses, or concentrate, or relax, without cigarettes; just as non-smokers do, in fact.

NRT, on the other hand, doesn't teach anyone anything. All it does is supply the substance to which smokers are addicted – nicotine – in a different way. Of course, patches, gums and lozenges are far less damaging than cigarettes, but nicotine replacement therapy doesn't 'replace' nicotine – it *is* nicotine … and there's certainly no therapy involved.

For the past 20 years or so, I've been sending clients wishing to stop smoking to the clinics run by Britain's internationally renowned quit smoking expert, Allen Carr. Allen has a remarkably high success rate in his worldwide network of clinics, and his famous book, *Allen Carr's Easy Way To Stop Smoking*, has sold over five million copies in 20 different languages.

Allen is completely opposed to NRT, arguing that you can't cure addicts by supplying them with the very substance to which they are addicted in the first place. He says smokers have been lured into the most subtle and ingenious trap imaginable, and it takes a little more expertise to free them from that trap than just dashing off a prescription for a nicotine patch, as so many hard-pressed GPs do. 'All substitutes make it more difficult to "give up" an addiction', Allen points out. 'That's because any substitute merely reinforces addicts' belief they are making a sacrifice. Even the expression "giving up" implies a sacrifice.'

Allen continues: 'Smokers suffer misery when they try to quit not because of physical withdrawal pains from nicotine, which are actually very slight, but because they believe they are being deprived of a genuine pleasure and/or crutch. Substitutes serve only to reinforce that deluded belief. Substitutes that contain nicotine have the added disadvantage of continuing the addiction to nicotine. I only ever refer to quitting or escaping cigarettes. Smoking is a disease! Ridding yourself of a disease is a cause for rejoicing, not feelings of deprivation.'

Allen himself was a 100-a-day smoker for more than 30 years, and tried repeatedly to give up before stumbling on a way of thinking about smoking and why he was doing it that helped him break free. Since then, he has dedicated his life to freeing other smokers, and I believe it's a public health scandal that the taxpayer-funded quit smoking authorities in this and other countries don't seek Allen's advice and guidance, as many major international private companies do.

As with so many other public health issues, though, the problem is that the quit smoking authorities are wedded to a medical-model approach. Because doctors are the leading experts on the damage to health that smoking does, most people assume this also makes them the experts on giving up. The pharmaceutical companies that make NRT products subtly play to this assumption, providing doctors with nicotine in a medicalized form which they can prescribe. In a single bound, nicotine goes from being the problem to the solution! Except that so many smokers remain hooked, even using NRT just to tide them over on those occasions when smoking is banned, such as on public transport and in restaurants.

The drug companies are also the only organizations rich enough to be able to mount the very expensive double-blind, randomized clinical trials that health authorities demand before they will endorse any method as 'clinically proven'. Never mind if clinical trials prove that NRT fails to help the overwhelming majority of smokers who use it – all that seems to matter to public health bureaucrats is that the trials have been conducted, regardless of the outcome.

Yet the mere fact that smokers are offered a substitute by their GPs helps reinforce their fear and panic that they are making some sort of terrible sacrifice in 'giving up' cigarettes. Allen, and other successful quit smoking therapists, by contrast, emphasize the positive – that quitting can be surprisingly easy, and that people should celebrate their release when they finally manage to break free of such an insidious and deluded addiction.

For more information on Allen Carr's Easyway method, visit www.allencarrseasyway.com or call 0800 389 2115.
For more information on NRT issues, visit www.whyquit.com.

Conclusion

It's not the case, as too many of us assume, that we are powerless as isolated individuals to resist the might of the mega-multinational pushers of junk food, junk chemicals and junk pharmaceutical drugs.

We *do* have the power, either as consumers choosing what we spend our money on, as voters or as campaign activists. We can make a difference to our own personal environment and quality of life. But we have to make the effort to seek out the information we need to make properly informed choices in the first place. Which means we have to get off our butts and get on with it!

Looking in the Mirror

2

NEVER UNDERESTIMATE HOW much your body is affected by your emotions. Being either happy, stressed, grief-stricken or scared changes every fibre, cell and reaction in your body. Present and past traumas are stored in the subconscious and can play a significant role in ill health, as well as in a person's ability to make a full recovery.

Our personalities are partly inherited from one or both of our parents. As babies and children we are deeply affected by childhood experiences, absorbing the feelings of everyone around us. Then there are the enormous influences of a culture that shapes the aspirations, requirements and implicit rules of life. Piece by piece, our brains construct the sense of identity we come to take for granted – who we are – along with myriad ways of seeing the world that determine our sense of pleasure and self-esteem, as well as our ability to adjust to and cope with life's difficulties.

Often our ability to create the situations and outcomes we want is spoilt by continuous unwanted patterns. This is why some of us seem to experience a *Groundhog Day* series of repetitive problems with work or relationships that never seem to last. We may have a nagging, pervasive sense of emptiness or a feeling that our lives are not complete and that things aren't right.

I Can Handle It

Whatever a child's negative emotions, they are quickly aired. Emotions are supposed to be like this – fleeting and transitory. The body temporarily shuts down some of its systems when adrenaline has been released, for instance, because adrenaline is only supposed to last long enough to help us run away from immediate danger.

As they grow up, children are restrained, disciplined, overpowered or suppressed. And, as a result, they can become self-conscious, embarrassed and fearful about expressing themselves. Natural honesty and freedom of action, motion and speech become stifled and altered. At school, we are programmed to take in academic information. We are not nearly so encouraged to understand and explore the personal and emotional areas of our lives. We are conditioned not to say or do things out of place. By early adulthood, we have learned to put up or shut up. As children, our bodies were our main barometer for how we felt, and we'd act accordingly. As adults, we access a great deal of emotional information via our brains. Thinking this is a way we can control outcomes, we build an emotional pain threshold which, for too many people, has no upper limit.

This can result in people putting up with less than satisfactory relationships, financial stresses or ongoing illnesses that erode their bodies year in, year out. The amount of emotional pain we learn to put up with can be more debilitating than anything else and is prevalent in contributing to the onset of major illness and depression. Ironically, spending time learning how to *lower* your emotional pain threshold can transform your health and your life. Maybe being able to 'handle it all' is not such a great success story after all.

Emotional Intelligence

At times there is a real need for some outside assistance when it comes to acquiring emotional intelligence. As well as helping your specific predicament, it is likely to make everyone's life around you a lot better too. The ability to see ourselves accurately is a skill in itself. Receiving constructive criticism, while rejecting any opinions about ourselves that are inaccurate or unjust, is a part of learning how to acquire self-knowledge. If you are someone who isn't afraid to challenge yourself, you can reach a point where more often than not satisfaction becomes the norm. It's not easy, but eventually you will find that anything that threatens your equilibrium will be incorporated in a constructive and, in time, a positive way. How you do it, though, is completely up to you.

If someone has tried everything to lose weight, or to address a more serious recurring health issue, they may well, without knowing it, be undermining their chances of success because of emotional issues. However, it can be very difficult to stand back and take a good look at oneself. This is not a skill we learn early in life, yet taking stock of your overall health, not just how you feel physically but how you feel emotionally too, is absolutely essential. Think of it as taking a personal inventory, both physically and emotionally. And yes, it does take time in a life which is probably overcharged anyway, but it can make all the difference to how quickly and easily you achieve your goal.

I have devised a questionnaire on www.lifesmart.co.uk for you to fill out, that will help you to open up your viewpoint in every direction and allow you to see the full picture. The questions will help you put together your own case history, enabling you to make the necessary connections between your physical background, state of mind and the way your body behaves. When you do go to see a doctor, complementary practitioner, counsellor, fitness expert or nutritionist, you will be able to brief them, ask pertinent questions and troubleshoot, allowing you to get the best out of them.

Personalities

Throughout our lives, we can find ourselves 'stuck' with aspects of our personality that keep us from reaching our full potential. If we are fortunate enough to become aware of this, we can deal with it and move on. Here are a handful of examples of characteristics that hinder growth and which you may well recognize in yourself or others close to you. For those of you who are well aware that some help would be advantageous the guide on pages 35–43 will be particularly relevant.

The Ego

A healthy measure of confidence goes a long way. But people who ignore the signs that they are crippling their bodies through their own self-indulgent habits, or who are reluctant to let go of a lifestyle that poses risks to their health, well-being, quality of life and relationships, often end up worse off for it. In truth, it's not much fun behind that façade, but when something manages to get under their skin, they usually come through with flying colours.

'Yes' People

There are two types of 'yes' people. The first type agree with everything that is suggested and are very 'nice'. They are the ones who insist sincerely that they are doing everything that they've been advised to do, but who mysteriously do not lose weight or feel any better. Unless a medical condition is diagnosed, they aren't actually telling those trying to help – or themselves – the truth. These people tend to yo-yo from one practitioner to another or do numerous mind and body therapies in tandem, never completing a course of action. Those who manage to get results often quickly revert to type and continue their ongoing quest to find the 'missing' answers, even though they have been given the answers already. When they are tackled directly it can be quite a shock to uncover a not so nice and cuddly person underneath.

The second type of yes people are those who look after everyone else rather than themselves. They are genuinely very nice, and are quick to adjust once they realize that if they take themselves in hand, everyone around them benefits.

The Non-believer

Not believing in anything is the ultimate get-out clause and excuse for never doing anything to change, or take any particular course of action. This character has already made the decision that nothing works, that they know better, using scientific terminology to back up their arguments... The non-believer has 'an answer' for everything.

The Smiley Person

Many people feel under pressure to keep up appearances. They make it their priority to not divulge what's really happening. Anyone caught in this trap is under constant strain and often insular, even if they appear sociable. They live their lives as if watching themselves on film. The purpose is to show the world that everything is all right. Addiction, covert behaviour and depression are common problems experienced by these characters.

The Flaky Person

This is someone who almost beats down the gym door to train; then, more often than not, ends up either cancelling or continually turning up late. They often make out they know a great deal about their bodies, but are in fact completely disconnected and oblivious to their impact on others. They speak a lot – anything that takes them as far away from concentrating on their own bodies as possible. Flaky people talk a good talk, sound like they know what they are doing about their diet or exercise regime, but rarely stick at it, being 'on the run' in every area of their lives. They can be terribly nice, admit to all their binges and lose a stone in weight – only to put it back on in a tenth of the time it took to lose it.

The NSD Person

NSD or Non-Specific Discontent seems to be the new malaise. You will recognize NSD in people who are always wishing that they were doing something else with their lives; they are constantly not having their needs met. Other people with NSD, who seemingly have everything, are moody, rude and condescending, especially to their partners and at work. Bitterness often creeps in and they always have a negative answer to any positive suggestions. Generosity is rare, especially when it comes to acknowledging the ideas and triumphs of others. Illness is a common occurrence, gradually eroding the body over a long period of time. This sort of character is probably tougher to crack than any of the other types, and one can only hope, if they do end up on a practitioner's doorstep, that he or she is strong enough to take them in hand.

None of these personality types is particularly problematic. But they serve as useful indicators of the traits that can stop us having the healthy, happy lives and bodies we purport to want to have. If you recognize yourself in any of these types and think you have taken steps to deal with the problems, but know in your heart that you are just plastering over the cracks, then you have to decide what is more important; maintaining the status quo, or being honest with yourself and moving forward.

The flip side of all of this is maybe you don't want to change. You may be one of those people who have had children, have financial security, an interesting group of friends, an active sex life, but yet is continually seeing 'shrinks' or doing multiple complementary therapies, and still remains dissatisfied. It's simply a matter of admitting that this is the way you like it. You're getting plenty of attention and you're not quite ready to admit that there is actually nothing wrong. That is fine as long as it doesn't get out of control, doesn't hurt other people, and you are honest about your motivations.

Fear Of Being Alone

We all have a natural inclination to panic about gaps, rushing in to fill what we perceive as 'vacuums'. So when we break up from a relationship, lose a loved one, or have to leave a job, our emotions can be unbearable. The sense of panic we feel when we walk alone into the yawning chasm of pubs, parties or restaurants has us wanting to tune out. You know the feeling when you are almost squirming inside from discomfort, embarrassment and/or shyness, and grab the nearest drink in order to blot it all out. In fact, when life treats us badly, as it invariably does, it can be an extraordinary time, a golden opportunity to catch up with oneself and make far-reaching decisions and substantial changes. If you don't know where to begin and can't get past the weepiness or feeling of desolation then some form of therapy can really help. Only too often, people are desperate to fill a gap and rush into another relationship or a new job before they have given themselves the luxury of time to heal and re-establish their own relationship with themselves.

So, Who Can Help You?

Becoming emotionally healthy and knowledgeable can be made a lot easier with help from outside. But it can be hard to find the answers to whom, where and how. You have to research it and also usually have to be prepared to pay a substantial amount of money, hence it is important not to rush into anything too hastily. Check what's available on the NHS and how long you would have to wait to see someone.

Unfortunately, a large number of professionals who work in this area want you to stay with them for years on end, some seeing you as often as three times per week, thereby diluting any sustainable independent result. Others want you to do their 'enlightenment courses' for the best part of the rest of your life.

It's not that you won't derive some benefit from both sets of people – for a period – but it only ever translates into something truly effective when you are no longer reliant on it and have moved on within a given period of time… A structured programme that involves a mix of approaches and a time frame – possibly starting on a one-to-one basis, and then finishing by attending a group course teaching specific skills and tools – can be an extremely effective way to proceed.

There's still a stigma, though, attached to seeking help. Most of us associate only serious depression, schizophrenia, or some sort of '-ism' (for instance, alcoholism) with the need to seek professional help. Otherwise, we assume we are admitting we are weak or not 'up to it'. And indeed, drugs or years of psychotherapy are still the mainstay of dealing with serious mental health or psychological problems. Yet traumas, phobias and learned – or unlearned – behaviour from our childhood can easily influence how, without knowing it, we either shut down or deal ineffectively with any conundrum that arises in our lives. We have no problem with being happy or satisfied, but we strongly resist learning how to manage apathy, fear, grief, anger and pride. Because we're not encouraged at an early age to move through these emotions, it is very hard, if not impossible, to see them as opportunities to gain wisdom and insight. Recognizing that life is essentially a series of crises and breakthroughs can transform the way you handle hardship.

Where to Get Help

One of the myths about getting help with emotional difficulties is that there are only two options – talking therapies, or taking drugs for a period of time. But that is not necessarily the case. Sometimes, a trauma manifests in such a way that the best approach for dealing with life's challenges is through more physical therapies: for example, meditation and visualization; hypnotherapy; acupuncture; or homeopathy, to mention just a few options.

Acupuncture, for instance, is to be recommended in an acute situation. If you can get yourself to the practitioner, the treatment will calm you down so that you are better able to decide on the next step. It's at that initial hysterical point that so often hits in the first 24 hours after an emotional shock, when a non-verbal interaction can be very constructive. Homeopathy can back up any action you take. I would always choose homeopathic medication rather than pharmaceutical drugs as they are powerful, effective and non-addictive, with no side effects

Floating Along

My colleagues and I often encounter people who have been 'in therapy' for many years – sometimes going up several times per week – but in truth feel that they have made little or no progress, only are too scared to tell the therapist. My advice is to take time out, either between individual sessions or every few weeks, to digest and apply what you've learnt, and also to take stock. The timing is different for every individual, because when you're starting out there is a natural need to follow a routine and not break the cycle of therapy too soon. Talk to your therapist about this – but be prepared to use your own judgment.

State as clearly as you can that you want to achieve tangible goals, eventually reducing the number of sessions and moving on. Analysts, therapists, gurus, facilitators – whatever you choose to call them – can be very seductive in keeping treatment or analysis going.

Conversely, be honest with yourself and don't stop seeing your therapist before you are well and truly ready.

Following are brief descriptions of the main cognitive and physical therapies available to you.

NLP

Neurolinguistic Programming – NLP – studies how our unique experiences of life and the world are created, maintained and changed. It starts from very simple premises and a number of tools for 'patterning' behaviour and can lead … well … almost anywhere you would care to go.

While it makes no claim to be scientific, NLP uses careful observation of body language, emotional states, awareness, language and mental processes such as beliefs and attitudes, to figure out what needs to happen in order for someone to change their behaviour, learn something new, or change how they feel. It has applications in therapy and counselling, sports motivation, business and any other area in life where people want to develop.

NLP was created in the 1970s by mathematician Richard Bandler and linguist John Grinder, both of whom were interested in studying and exploring the implications of language and non-verbal behaviour during effective therapy. They studied the behaviour of many 'greats' in the field of therapy at that time and, as their studies spread to other disciplines, they discovered that success always leaves clues. From their work, the discipline of NLP was born.

If you've heard about NLP but not experienced it, you might have the idea that it uses lots of jargon and strange-sounding labels. You can, however, take what you need from it and set the rest aside.

One of the most practical uses of Neurolinguistic Programming is in any relationship, either personal or work, where, by using its tools, you can learn to understand someone else's point of view and how they are feeling – without having to impose your own views on to them. Learning to communicate your needs more effectively and how to alter your own negative reactions and interpretations are just a couple of areas NLP concentrates on. The purpose is to be very practical and help individuals and groups to get the best out of themselves and each other.

For more information see www.purenlp.com/society.htm.

Hypnotherapy/Hypno-psychotherapy

Hypnosis – from the Greek word to 'sleep' – is a state of heightened awareness or altered consciousness achieved by means of verbal suggestion by a hypnotist. This state can be used to manipulate the perception of pain, to access repressed material and to change behaviour. The degree of hypnotic state may vary from mild increased suggestibility to that comparable to anaesthesia.

Hypnotherapy has been used for centuries, and in the 1800s hypnosis was widely practised by physicians, who used it both as an anaesthetic and analgesic before drugs, as we now know them, existed.

Although psychoanalysis and psychotherapy have been used as alternatives, hypnotherapy remains a popular and adaptive tool for anything from simple relaxation therapy to helping treat depression. Today there is also a combination of hypnotherapy and psychotherapy, and this integrative approach is termed hypno-psychotherapy.

Complex emotional, psychological or physical problems require the help of a fully qualified and experienced hypno-psychotherapist. Addictive behaviours, lack of confidence, phobias and insomnia are also treatable, and hypnotherapy has been successfully used for enhancing memory, concentration and performance in sports and tests.

Hypnotherapy is used as a tool across a spectrum of training and self-help approaches, such as NLP. Some people swear by hypnotherapy. Many people who are very cynical about hypnotherapy but try it are often surprised by its effectiveness. There are others who, without being judgmental or negative, simply don't respond at all. If you are someone who can be put in a deep meditative state through breathing and visualization, you can access behavioural and attitudinal changes in a far-reaching way. Many hypnotherapists will teach you how to practise taking yourself to this state, as well as giving you a relaxation tape or CD to enhance that. This is usually how the best long-term results are attained.

For more information call the hypnotherapy register on 01590 683 770.

Life Coaching

Coaching – often preceded by the word 'life' – seems to have sprung up from nowhere to be, quite literally, everywhere. Television programmes such as *Changing Rooms* and *Ground Force* offer a quick fix for your home or garden; life coaches, or life gurus, are portrayed as offering an equally quick fix for your 'life' problems. This is not a true representation of what practical life coaching is all about.

It is worth looking beyond the apparent instant gratification aspect of coaching to see where it has come from, what it has to offer, and what it may be able to do for you. While coaching has its roots in the world of sports, it first made its appearance in the business world around 10–15 years ago. The idea of having a secure job for life had virtually disappeared, and with this came a requirement to be more flexible, to be able to accept change, to adapt and to take responsibility for one's own life.

People from a wide range of professions and walks of life started coaching other people for a fee and the audience widened. At one end of the scale, there are coaches whose children have left home and who are now keen to pass on the advice they used to give to their offspring – an approach very similar to 'agony aunting'. At the other end are the famous self-help gurus who will step down from the motivational speaker's stage and work with you one-to-one (some for an extremely large fee).

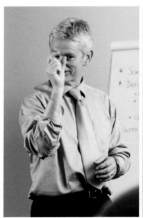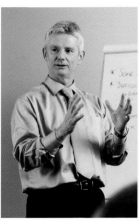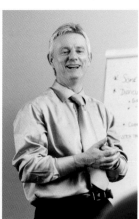

Mike Duckett, life coach, in action. Mike has a corporate background but is also a trained psychotherapist – a rare and very useful combination for a life coach.

Many people – including those formerly known as therapists – rebranded themselves as life coaches. Trainers and business consultants also marketed themselves as executive coaches. Whether or not they make a successful transition depends very much on their attitude to the client. They can see their client either as someone who is setting out to achieve a goal, or as someone who has a problem that needs sorting out.

Executive coaching is usually targeted towards improving performance at work. It is likely to have as its starting point the need to develop better managerial or motivational abilities, for example for a manager to become a more charismatic leader or to improve presentation skills.

In some cases, I suspect coaching is seen as a way of rejuvenating training and business consultancies with a trendier label – while at the same time opening up an additional revenue stream. In fact, all the large consultancies now offer executive coaching, as does the Institute of Directors, because when done well it can be an extremely effective (and cost-effective) method of management development.

Traditional therapy is problem-centered. It is often said that therapy looks backwards and dwells on the question of why things are as they are, which means the conversation will focus the client very much on the current situation and only then move on to explore the options for moving forward.

Coaches, on the other hand, take a completely different view. As one coach said to me: 'People can sit down and discuss what is happening in their life and all their problems in great depth, because this is all very familiar. As a coach, your job is not to let them dwell on this. You need to move them along by asking them what they want to achieve. When they start to think about that, they've immediately begun to make progress.'

The role of the coach is therefore to help clients to clarify and define their goals, to challenge their conventional thinking, to stimulate, encourage, provide feedback (both positive and negative) and support them in achieving their aims.

For more information see www.coachingforsuccess.co.uk
or www.coachfederation.org

HeartMath

HeartMath is a highly effective, innovative system of stress reduction and performance enhancement based on recent breakthroughs in scientific knowledge about the workings of the heart, brain and central nervous system. Tapping into a mass of recent research showing how our emotions and feelings both affect and are affected by our heart rhythms, HeartMath blends neuroscience, cardiology, psychology, physiology, biochemistry and physics.

All strong emotions affect the pattern of our heart rhythms. When people are frustrated, scared, worried, angry or upset, their heartbeat is jagged, uneven and irregular. When people are happy, confident and secure, on the other hand, their heart rate is smooth, ordered and regular. And because the heart, brain and emotions are all interconnected, smooth and even heart rhythms make it far easier for people to think clearly and calmly and control their emotions.

The human heart is more than a muscle. Years ago, scientists discovered that it also contains its own nervous system, comprising some 40,000 neurons, or nerve cells. In other words, the heart has its own 'mini-brain', which communicates directly with the primary brain's 100 billion neurons.

The different aspects of the brain

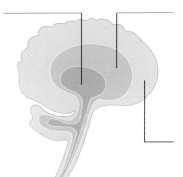

1st Brain: Reflex/Instinct
Functions and basic drives:
- Approach/avoidance
- Hormonal control
- Temperature control
- Hunger/thirst
- Reproductive drive
- Respiration and heart
  rate control

2nd Brain: Hindsight
Functions and basic drives:
- Territoriality
- Fear
- Anger
- Maternal love
- Social bonding
- Jealousy

3rd Brain: Foresight
Functions and basic drives:
- Self-awareness of
  thoughts and emotions
- Ability to choose
  appropriate behaviour
- Self-reflection
- Goal satisfaction

How heart activity affects how we feel

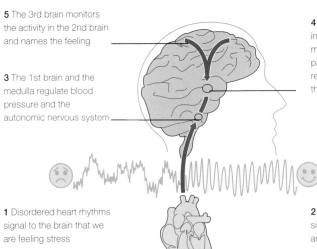

5 The 3rd brain monitors the activity in the 2nd brain and names the feeling

3 The 1st brain and the medulla regulate blood pressure and the autonomic nervous system

4 The 2nd brain (which includes the amygdala) monitors heart rhythm patterns and other body responses to sense how the body is feeling

1 Disordered heart rhythms signal to the brain that we are feeling stress

2 Ordered heart rhythms signal to the brain that we are feeling calm and positive

Emotions affect perceptions; perceptions affect emotions; and both affect and are affected by the heart's signals to and from the brain via the autonomic nervous system. That's why, for example, constant feelings of anger and stress can lead to high blood pressure and even heart attacks.

Do we experience happiness, contentment and other positive emotions randomly, entirely outside our control, or can we choose to create these beneficial feelings? HeartMath believes that with practice, we can learn to control our heart rhythms and thereby take charge of our emotions, whatever is happening to us externally. To begin with, HeartMath techniques help people manage minor irritations, anxieties or anger. With practice, though, they can ensure healthy heart rhythm patterns even during the most crushing disasters and worries.

As such, this technique has three main uses – combating physical health problems such as high blood pressure and heart disease; significantly improving learning and behaviour in classrooms, including helping children with ADD and ADHD; and improving performances under stressful conditions.

Created by an American called Doc Childre, a pioneer in the field of stress research, HeartMath techniques are now taught in schools, hospitals and government organizations throughout the US, as well as in many major international corporations such as BP, Unilever and HSBC.

For more information, go to www.heartmath.org.
To contact HeartMath's British representatives, Hunter Kane Ltd, visit www.hunterkane.com or call 01189 890 101.

Large Group Analysis Methods

Large Group Analysis Methods began with Werner Erhard and his est seminars in America over 30 years ago. Est has a view on human beings and how they behave which draws extensively on behavioural psychology, over-simplified Zen, crowd psychology and American show business.

Est (now known as the Forum), Silver Mind and similar methods such as the now-defunct Exegesis use a subtle form of hypnotic mind suggestion plus spiritualism on large groups of people at one time. These methods arose out of the desire – very popular in the 1960s and 1970s – to create a Western-style approach to consciousness-raising, as opposed to Eastern ways such as meditation and mantras.

Some people who have undergone such courses insist that they give helpful insights, philosophies and world views of what appropriate behaviour and emotional life should 'look' and feel like. Other people consider them to be evil, mind-bending cults. The truth is probably somewhere in the middle.

What is clear, however, is that these courses concentrate on 'de-programming' people to help them think in a new way. As a result, they tend to attract many people who are dysfunctional and vulnerable, with masks of arrogance or timidity. This approach is usually traumatic and exaggerated, and often is extremely irritating for the loved ones of participants. Until these trainings and their mentors are 'broken down' themselves, the assistance you seek may be better gained through other self-help therapies.

Psychotherapists

Psychotherapists were originally purveyors of the so-called 'talking' cure. Also known as psychoanalysts or in slang terms 'shrinks', these therapists are the modern-day disciples of Freud, Jung and others of that ilk.

The methods used include analytical therapy, behavioural therapy and existential therapy. Unfortunately, all of these methods can take years and are generally expensive.

Make sure that you discuss what kind of method or methods your psychotherapist is planning to use, and also find out how long they think the therapy will last for. Some clients have told me that their psychotherapists have been disapproving or even threatening when they (the patients) decided it was time to close the chapter and move on.

Cognitive Therapists

Cognitive therapists concentrate on helping a person to reframe their reactions to a current problem or perception. This current mode has proved both popular and effective as it is relatively simple and does not rely on long-term attendance. Instead, you take the time to digest the work put into your sessions, fit it into your life, then see if and what still needs working on. It's very important to find a therapist you are not awestruck by, yet at the same time a person whom you can respect and trust.

When my mother Sylvia suffered a fire in her home a year ago she went into complete shock which manifested in a physical breakdown. Because she is used to dealing with other people in this state, she realized she needed professional input and called on cognitive therapist Ron Bracey to work her through the trauma. It was incredibly fast and effective and surprisingly subtle. Ron is one of the new breed of workers in this field and has done extensive training.

Clinical psychologists

Clinical psychologists work in various ways with patients who have emotional, behavioural and/or personality disorders of some sort. Specializations include occupational psychology, child psychology and sports psychology.

Counsellors

Counsellors are trained to interfere less in a patient's process than psychotherapists, as the counselling paradigm is based on the notion that all individuals need is a reflective listener. Rather than suggest or even tell clients what to do, counsellors ask questions and help clients reach their own conclusions. This can be lengthy and for some people frustrating; others appreciate the space that is given to them. Talking out loud, in a safe environment, to a relatively complete stranger, enables people to liberate themselves and therefore reach conclusions.

EMDR

Eye Movement Desensitizing and Reprocessing (EMDR) is an information-processing therapy. An eight-phase approach is used to rectify an existing condition or problem, which includes taking a complete history, preparing the client, identifying targets and their components, actively processing past, present and future aspects, and on-going evaluation. During EMDR the client attends to emotionally disturbing material in brief, sequential doses while simultaneously focusing on an external stimuli such as therapist-directed eye movements. After each set of movements the client briefly describes what he or she has experienced, and is taught techniques by the technician so that he or she can leave the session feeling in control and empowered. After successful treatment with EMDR therapy, previously disturbing memories and present situations should no longer be problematic, distress is relieved and negative beliefs are reformulated.

For more information see www.healthyplace.com.

BEST

The Bio Energetic Synchronization Technique (BEST) was devised by one-time chiropractor Dr Ted Mortar. He believes that the body heals in order of priority, and that when emotional blocks are removed the rest of the body can fully repair. Emotional stress, breathing, nutritional status, exercise and quality of rest are all key elements examined during BEST therapy.

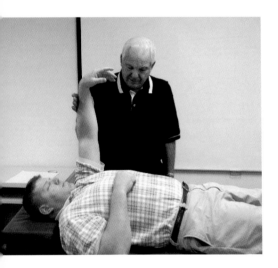

BEST (Bio-Energetic Synchronization Technique) was devised by one-time chiropractor Dr Ted Mortar.

I have included BEST because I have seen it achieve direct results in people who are emotionally paralyzed or who can't get rid of a physical condition or addiction. BEST has proved extremely effective for people with physical ailments, most commonly back problems and illnesses associated with the nervous system.

BEST works in the following way. Having suggested a word to concentrate on that is pertinent to the client, the practitioner puts his or her finger on a sensitive area of the body, particularly the cranium, while the client concentrates on that word, holding their breath and focusing their eyes in a direction, as instructed. This is repeated until all painful sensation has disappeared. At first you may only notice a slight feeling of 'lightness' in the body. However, it's quite likely a marked shift will be noticed physiologically and emotionally. After subsequent sessions you may feel that your symptoms and emotions have noticeably lifted, and that your physical ailments have disappeared.

For more information see www.mortar.com

Shamanism

The philosophy behind shamanism is that each individual can learn how to use the wisdom of nature and the elements to overcome obstacles. Shamanism hones each person's intuition, confidence and ability to guide themselves through life. Shamanic teachers have no fixed dogma or religion. They believe that every element of our environment and the events in our life can be called upon to teach and support, providing guidance in obtaining and maintaining health and emotional equilibrium. They believe we all have an innate intelligence based on intuition and instinct that can be retrieved and used to teach vital survival techniques. Shamans teach a working meditation that can help people overcome hysteria, acute fear, or any other emotion or problem.

This method is incredibly effective and attracts very academically inclined people. It has also been known to have far-reaching effects with seriously troubled teenagers and addicts.

As the emphasis is on the natural environment, Shamanism often takes a quite physical approach, including outdoor retreats and vision quests. The many different ways Shamans work include combinations of lectures and discussions, role playing, mental and physical exercises, demonstrations and videos.

Doing The Ground Work

CASE STUDY – TRAINING COURSES

Camille Squire is in her twenties and works in sales and marketing as a successful manager. She decided that she wanted to add some new skills in order to take on bigger challenges and manage her team more effectively. She chose an open public training course which lasted a week at a cost of two thousand pounds with 350 attendees. This particular course appealed to her because the three master trainers had a formidable reputation – she was expecting great things from it. Initially, she enjoyed the training, but after a couple of days began to feel cheated. One trainer she felt was just a showman, constantly whipping up the crowd and performing tricks. Another had a very uncomfortable body image and seemed to compensate by being incredibly 'charismatic and cool', using his size to show off, but conversely refrained from fully making eye contact with anyone. The third one, who devised the training, was extremely rude and dismissive. Camille readily admitted that there seemed to be many people on the course who benefited hugely and raved about their week. Whereas others like her felt let down.

So, was this training a rip-off or was Camille and the other disappointed trainees closed and judgmental? The answer is neither. Over the past 20 years I have come across many similar trainers. The majority have a vast amount of useful information, however they can often exhibit many irritating and dysfunctional characteristics. Not every training is suitable for everyone. Some programmes will suit certain types more than others.

You can't go into any self-learning situation with rose tinted glasses on, neither will you get any benefit from being uptight or cynical. Everyone has flaws and weaknesses. Some of the best teachers, therapists and trainers have the biggest problems and challenges themselves, which is why they are often very gifted in the work that they do. At present, there isn't an adequate screening process for trainings, but the information that you can glean, and take away with you, can be very valuable.

To find a good trainer you have to do your research. Ask about the format and subject matter of the course and how that is broken down. Use all the resources available, including websites and talking to other people. Personally I don't think any group training course should have more than 50 people. Whether it is one-to-one or group trainings you need to be sure that it fits with your requirements as best you can. And on your side, whatever you end up doing, it helps to put in 100 per cent.

There are some excellent individuals and companies who seem to strike exactly the right balance in the information they impart and how it's delivered. For example, Harvest is a small company run by a married couple with two children. They work mainly with small groups (no more than 15 people) and one-to-one with managers and directors. While being very successful, they have not developed over-inflated egos and the key to their accomplishments is that they don't try to make the individuals, companies or groups of people fit their training. Even if they get a brief from a boss, they spend a day getting to know each person and what their needs are. As a result, participants come away feeling satisfied without needing a crutch or further input.

Communication Skills Training

Everything up until now has largely been to do with understanding and reframing our negative thoughts, thereby changing our patterns and behaviour. One aspect that is not encompassed in the above choices, and is only touched on in NLP, are specific skills to do with verbal and non-verbal communication, listening skills, trouble shooting, body language, voice tone and motivation skills.

Businesses in the UK and abroad have been providing this training for the last 25 years, and the vast majority of participants report they get enormous value that positively affects every area of their lives and relationships. The core emphasis of this training method is to educate people to elicit cooperation and understanding from others. NLP is often incorporated as well, as the rapport skills it teaches are a key factor in defusing hostility and creating and promoting a positive response.

A beneficial side effect of this type of training is that it helps people not to be led by the emotion of a situation, but promotes listening on both sides with the desire to come to a win-win solution.

For more information and other associations, email: info@harvesttraining.com or call 0117 930 8888.

Alcoholics Anonymous (AA)

One area that is being acknowledged more than ever before is addiction. While there are rehabilitation services, both outpatients and residential, they are relatively exclusive both in terms of being very expensive and taking up an immense amount of time. The majority of people have neither. In terms of tangible results, there is also still great debate as to how much they help.

Alcoholics Anonymous (AA) began in Ohio in 1935 as the outcome of a meeting between a distinguished surgeon and a New York stockbroker, both severe alcoholics. After three initial years of trial and error in selecting the most workable tenets on which the new fellowship could be based, and after a large amount of failure in getting alcoholics to recover, three successful local groups emerged. The infant society set down its experiences in a book called *Alcoholics Anonymous*, from which it took its name.

• One in 13 people in the UK is dependent on alcohol, twice as many as the number of people hooked on all forms of drugs, legal and illegal.

The basic principles were borrowed mainly from religion and medicine, but many of the ideas in practice today were the result of noting the behaviour and needs of participants themselves. It was out of this experience that AA's famous Twelve Step programme, first codified in 1946, took form. Now there have been similar associations set up for almost every type of addiction, from food to sex.

AA and its related associations are non-profit organizations and are seen as the mother and father of all self-help programmes. It's said that if doctors could bottle what it offers, they would. The AA manages to maintain complete and total confidentiality that even the media cannot corrode, which is quite astonishing considering the number of celebrities, entrepreneurs and politicians who attend meetings. These associations don't profess to solve all your problems, but they offer a way to help you to take responsibility, gain an understanding of your addiction and progress to functional living.

CASE STUDY – REFLECTIONS OF AN AA CLIENT

I didn't get drunk every day. I didn't even get drunk every time I had a drink (though most times I did). I didn't always do something wrong, shameful or embarrassing each time (though most times I did). But, when I did have a drink, I never knew where it would take me. Once I had alcohol in me I ceased to be the master of my life and anything could happen. I might turn up for a meeting – I might not. I might promise not to have too many (what did that mean – too many for you or too many for me?). On the other hand I might not promise anything. I might be caring and faithful – or I might not...

Alcohol was the rocket fuel that propelled me through late adolescence and early adulthood. Without it I would never have coped with my social awkwardness, my loneliness, my fear of so many things, my guilt, my lack of self-worth, my deep-seated discontent and my unhappiness.

But somewhere, somehow, alcohol stopped being the solution and turned into the problem. My life became a morass of broken promises, lost friendships, self-hurt, humiliation, abuse and despair. I became locked in a raging anger against all and everyone, hurt the people I loved the most and allowed others to mistreat me. Yet, while I plunged deeper and deeper into the world of sordid places I resolutely judged others for their shortcomings and lack of moral fibre.

I didn't choose to seek out AA. The last thing I wanted to do was to stop drinking. All I wanted to do was to get the buzz back – for alcohol to do again what it once did. I just wanted alcohol to start fixing me again. And to achieve that I tried again and again to drink, regardless of the unpredictable, but increasingly disastrous, consequences.

So I didn't choose AA – I was taken to my first meeting by my long-suffering partner of the time. I went for a few months – anything for some peace and quiet – and I carried on drinking. And the consequences? They just kept getting worse and the feelings of despair intensified. Finally, early one morning, I hit rock bottom and realized that I couldn't go on any more with the consequences of my drinking. I just didn't know how to stop. That was the morning that I received the gift of desperation and finally asked for help. I reached out to someone I knew in AA and on that day I started my road to recovery.

Thirteen years on, I have not had to have a drink again in order to face life. Today life is not something to be endured but a daily journey (sometimes difficult, mostly not) filled with new discoveries, cherished old friends and bridges to family members that I had hurt. I have tried to right past wrongs where possible. I try to live my life to the full, taking care to avoid hurting those who come into contact with me. I enjoy a busy and very challenging career, a reasonable social life and friendships with many wonderful people both inside and outside AA. I happily give of my time to AA – working with newcomers – attempting to pass on something of the wisdom that was freely given to me.

Before I go to bed each night I take account of what has happened in my day. I gratefully conclude that I have been brought back from the pits of hopelessness and granted a second chance to have a good life. Today, with the help of AA, I plan to keep making good that chance.

• Death rates from alcohol-related diseases among 25- to 44-year-olds have trebled in the past 20 years, while 65 per cent of all suicides are alcohol-related.

Tough Love

So far, I have largely concentrated on therapies that address areas of personal dysfunction. The other side to this is when we find ourselves in a situation with loved ones where *their behaviour* is destructive both to themselves and those around them; when they are aggressive and often dangerous. Most of us try to cope on our own and overcompensate for the other person, especially where children are concerned. Without knowing it our fuse becomes shorter and shorter, but in order to handle the situation our pain thresholds expand. We start off trying to placate or please the other person into more rational behaviour, and when that doesn't work we may close up and stop communication altogether. Far more commonly, we get drawn into explosive arguments, constant screaming and shouting which – without us knowing – is exactly what that type of personality thrives on. Alcoholics Anonymous call this 'enabling'.

This situation can go on for years. It is imperative, even if you think you may be wrong, to find out what you're actually dealing with. It's a good idea for you to talk to somebody, just to limit the damage and erosion that undoubtedly will be occurring within your heart and head, so you can come through this as unscathed as possible. Your GP should be a good source of information and advice, and there are many associations on the web that will give you information, plus guidelines of where you can go to get help face-to-face. One of the best sources of information and support for enlightening you as to the tell-tale signs, the problems and the courses of action available to you is the AA-related organization Al-Anon (see page 221).

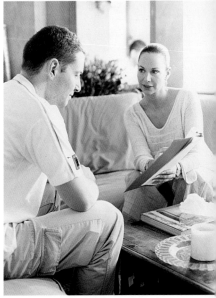

A typical LifeSmart consultation. We look at the bigger picture to see what combination of actions an individual may need to take to get consistent, long-lasting results.

More than any other problem discussed in this chapter, this situation highlights the importance of beginning to incorporate personal education about emotional health and functioning, both for ourselves and in relationship to everybody in our lives.

The Honeymoon Period – And When It's Over

When we've decided that we need to make an adjustment in our lives, nine times out of 10, there's an initial positive surge. This is because you are doing what works, in order of priority, in several areas at the same time. The first pitfall is that we take our early achievements for granted, or we become complacent, and so ends the honeymoon period. Emotional lows and highs further divert attention. These body-brain triggers start the self-sabotaging off again, and old habits re-emerge. Very quickly the mind descends towards: 'It's never going to work, what's the point' or 'I don't have the will-power to stick to this'. Feeling resentment, negativity and disappointment, before you know it you are, unfortunately, right back at square one.

But if you can look optimistically at what you have achieved to date, and, being realistic, understand that you have only gone off the rails for a short time, you don't need to feel guilty – just get straight back up again. I have an expression for it. I call it army drill. When I'm exhausted, migrainy, spotty, puffy and piling on a few pounds – all of which I'm easily susceptible to – instead of running around trying to get other people to piece me back together again, I take time out to see what needs to be dealt with first. Usually it's my emotional state, followed by lack of sleep and not eating sensibly. Get that in control, slow down your work and social life and take it from there. You will always have two voices in your head competing for your attention, one negative and one positive. It all depends on which one you allow to outshout the other.

Knowing Yourself

The brain has to be exercised just like any other part of your body. Will-power, strength of mind and discipline don't just decide to wing their way into your psyche – they have to be practised and cultivated like any other skill. It only takes a few seconds to remind yourself that the negative emotion, whatever it is, does not have to result in comfort eating, drinking or taking drugs. Don't be tempted to return to your old habits and 'cheer yourself up' after a temporary lapse.

Allowing disappointment and rejection to be part of your self-knowledge will always bring about a positive outcome, because you are learning to readjust how your mind views negative feelings and experiences. The trick of being successful in life is learning how to deal with the setbacks and problems that come your way, rather than using them as an excuse to undermine your health and well-being – which brings us to one of our favourite excuses.

Stress

It's amazing how some people can cope with immense stress and pressure, while others feel overwhelmed by the slightest change to their routine. Some people get anxious very easily, while others actively seek the thrills and sense of exhilaration that anxiety and uncertainty can bring.

We all know that there is good and bad stress, and that stress can be successfully used as a catalyst for growth and change. However, stress has become the catch-all excuse for not doing what you know you need to do, or for remaining in a rut. 'If only I wasn't so stressed, I would have the energy to cook better/eat better/go to the gym/pay my partner more attention/spend more time with the kids…'

• 13 million working days are lost each year due to stress. The cost to British companies is approximately £3.7 billion per year.

When we don't deal with stress, the body at first tries to regulate itself, using the hormonal system to limit the consequences. If nothing changes, physical symptoms start occurring to warn us that we are close to our limits. We override that warning system at our peril, as real damage sets in. There's a host of what we now know as stress-related illnesses: depression, insomnia, fatigue, irritability, poor digestion, muscle tension, high blood pressure, diabetes, heart problems – the list goes on. Because of the constant fatigue, you suffer the added burden of your brain distorting and exaggerating every little thing. A body under constant attack from stress suffers a great deal of wear and tear.

Tobacco, alcohol, caffeine, sugar and drug dependencies are all a feature of a stressed existence. It's no coincidence that the 'diehards' who thrash themselves daily in the gym or through sport will use one or more of these substances within half an hour of their session. I often watch people light up a cigarette as they walk out of the gym. Yet these damaging crutches just exacerbate the condition of the body's already beleaguered systems and organs. Giving them up will help you deal far more successfully and productively with stressful times. Every practitioner I have ever spoken to confirms that clients protest loudest and lie most about giving up their addictions. If only they would understand that nicotine, alcohol and drugs only serve to make stress harder – not easier – to deal with.

Many of you may not even be able to imagine a life where you aren't stressed or living in fear of everything coming crashing down around you. But it doesn't have to be this way. Physically and emotionally, there are several options available to you.

Ways of lowering stress naturally include: gentle exercise, herb and vitamin supplements, and various forms of complementary medicine such as homeopathy, acupuncture and massage. Acupuncture can be used for balancing the meridians and slowing down the physical adrenaline surge. Deep tissue massage followed by Reiki can reduce the build-up of muscle tension and relieve lymphatic blockage that can be caused by stress. Bathing at night, just before bed, helps calm the mind and body and promote better sleep.

Yet most people ignore the warning signs and continue to override their system until it can no longer cope. For many, it usually takes a complete collapse before they take steps to deal with the stress and habits that are compromising their systems. The key to survival is learning how to deal with, alleviate, make use of and learn from stress – *before* you fall flat on your face.

Conclusion

Changing how we react and how we deal with what life throws at us is tough. There are two factors that will make the difference between a successful result or a failure. They are firstly choosing the right method or person to help you, and secondly you yourself.

Many years ago, a wise person told me that the reactions I have to people and situations will tell me much more about me than it will about them.

However, it's not about getting rid of your existing personality, nor will you necessarily break every bad habit or pattern you have. You may not learn your lessons first time around, but if you are determined and courageous enough – constantly reminding yourself that less is more in terms of expectations, attention seeking and high drama – the rewards will far outweigh the negatives.

At the end of it all, you may find yourself feeling like Dorothy at the end of *The Wizard of Oz*. What you actually need has been with you from the beginning, but you simply didn't know how to recognize it. What if Dorothy had had to pay money at every stage of the way to the Scarecrow, Lion, Tin Man, Good Witch, Wicked Witch and the Wizard himself, only to discover at the end that she did not need any of these people, but could have gone home any time she wanted to, just by clicking her heels?

The changes that we want to make will always be inside of ourselves, but what it's going to take to learn to click our heels three times may be different for each one of us. In the end it comes down to a personal choice, often kick-started by admitting that we all need emotional intelligence in our lives to attain the real satisfaction and happiness that is readily available.

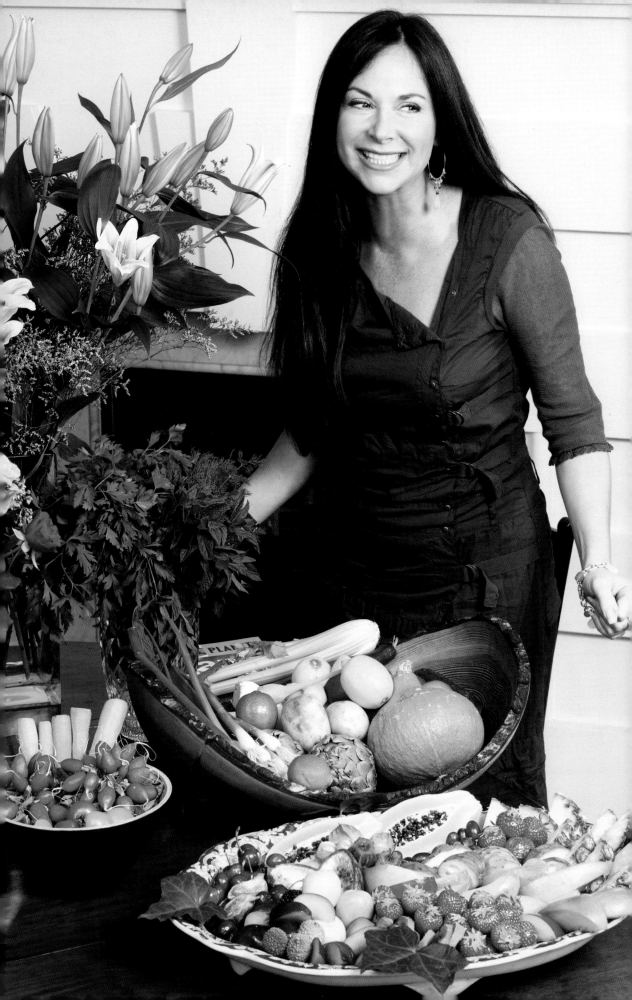

MAIN COURSE
EVOLVE YOUR IDEAS

Outside the Box

GETTING WELL REQUIRES KNOWING what resources are available to you on both sides of the medical fence – orthodox and complementary. Being dismissive of either approach simply denies your body the benefits of all available choices and know-how. Finding out about both the possibilities and limitations of each of these areas will help to stop the often never-ending cycle of recurring multiple illness building on top of one another and will hugely increase the chances of a positive final outcome.

More often than not, many of our daily malaises and illnesses can be cleared up through changes in nutrition, lifestyle and exercise levels – up to 75 per cent of people's troubles and symptoms can be resolved in this way. More serious health dilemmas, however, do need to be addressed by taking the time to look at the bigger picture. Think about managing your health as you would any other area of life such as your job, home and finances. In each of these areas, you are constantly evaluating the state of your affairs, prioritizing needs, anticipating difficulties and attempting to solve problems before they develop into a crisis – or at least, you should be. And your health is no different.

In a medical emergency, orthodox diagnosis and immediate treatment is clearly needed. However, once you are over the initial hurdle or left with any symptoms that are lingering or chronic, complementary therapies and alternative testing can often bring about lasting improvements without the side effects of prescription drugs and/or powerful painkillers.

It's not a question, as it is so often painted, of right or wrong. The emphasis is on doing what works for you and eliminating what doesn't. Then, if something does happen to your body, you are in the best position to deal with it.

No one person, regime or method, whether it be orthodox or complementary, is going to fit all of your requirements, match all of your expectations, or resolve all of your symptoms, especially over the course of your lifetime. For all the scaremongering and mud-slinging, there is a place for most schools of thought.

The reality is that any number of choices can irritate you, be contradictory or cause confusion. That's the nature of living. It doesn't mean that they don't contain any validity. The fundamental issue is not about how orthodox and complementary approaches differ, but how they can complete each other and work together or separately to achieve the best possible result.

Joanna's case history illustrates this. For many years, she had to struggle and search for answers. She received huge benefits from following an orthodox procedure that created a turning point for her, but the rest of her recovery came through a complementary approach. Most importantly, her story illustrates the difficulties, frustrations, values and benefits that so many people experience when trying to resolve health issues.

Joanna's journey, however, was needlessly long because she had to work it out for herself, often completely in the dark. Unfortunately, this is not a minority experience, but is happening to many people, often resulting in multiple, acute and chronic conditions on top of the initial problem.

CASE STUDY – JOANNA'S STORY

Ten years on, I am finally feeling as though I can see the end of the tunnel. It has not been an easy process and there has not been a clear path, which is perhaps why it has taken so long. At one point, I thought it was perhaps my fault that the doctors and specialists couldn't provide me with any answers. A few of them even suggested that was the case. I needed to handle my stress better. Toughen up a bit. All women have menstrual pain. And so on.

But I knew deep down there really was something wrong. It didn't take a genius to deduce that it wasn't normal to have regular rectal bleeding at the age of 17, and that despite a barium enema, colonoscopy, stool analysis and doctor's examination all showing no problems, this was not simply a case of me needing to eat more fibre and not stress over the ups and downs of first love. I also knew, despite my doctor's advice that it was 'safe' to take up to 16 Ibuprofen capsules a day (which I did for several days a month for nearly two years), that I needed to come up with a better long-term solution to debilitating menstrual cramps.

In the meantime, I continued to see my GP for the bowel issues and a gynaecologist for the menstrual pain. The two problems would not be linked until several years later – long after I had passed out at work from a particularly horrendous period, four years after I started taking the Pill to 'control' menstrual irregularities, and two years into being unable to have regular intercourse due to pain. At this point, after over six years with no clear answers, I gave up going to the doctor because I found it frustrating, humiliating and depressing.

Unfortunately, about this time the birth control pills were no longer able to mask that my body was in crisis. I was experiencing cramps three weeks of each month and rectal bleeding almost daily. I was exhausted. I would get up, go to work, sleep through my lunch hour with my head on my desk, work for a few more hours, go home and sleep from 5–8pm, get up to eat dinner with my husband and go back to bed. This went on for months. The bloating in my abdominal area fluctuated so much that I could wear three different trouser sizes in one month.

Then, a friend told me she had been diagnosed with endometriosis. As she told me more about the symptoms, it all started making sense. I spent the next few months on the internet learning everything I could about endometriosis: what it is, the symptoms, its connection with bowel issues, how it is treated, the prognosis and so on. I also researched the top reproductive endocrinologists and made an appointment with one of the best laparoscopic surgeons in the US.

I can remember the huge relief when he said that it was most likely that I did have endometriosis and that it seemed surgery would be my best option. As I drove away, I had to pull the car over as tears streamed down my face. Finally, I was going to get some answers. Finally, someone understood that I wasn't a wimp. Finally, I was going to get this sorted out.

At that time, I had a very naïve but common view of surgery as the ultimate problem solver. What could be more effective than a highly trained surgeon going right to the location of the problem?

I quickly learned it wasn't that simple. The surgery was a huge success, the specialist told me, but the endometriosis was chronic and would return. The plan now was to manage its re-growth and preserve my fertility. It turned out that we had not gone to the root of the problem at all – just merely scraped the evidence and symptoms away.

The surgeon then advised me that, at 23, my best chances of conceiving a child were in the next two years. Never mind that I hadn't dreamed of having children before 30, he assured me that there was 'never a perfect time to have kids'. If I wanted to wait longer, my best option was to take the Pill continuously for four months at a time, allowing my body to menstruate only three times per year and thus limiting the endometriosis re-growth. Then, if I couldn't conceive naturally, I could try IVF.

I left shocked and angry. I knew that statistically he was right about my chances of conception, but I couldn't believe the complete disregard for other areas of my life. I got back on the internet and started researching how I could deal with my endometriosis for the next 30 years until I hit menopause.

The internet provided a scary and depressing glimpse into a world of dismal statistics and message boards of women who felt disempowered and overwhelmed. It seemed the vast majority of prescription alternatives for women in my position, or at the next stage of going through fertility treatments, came with a lot of side effects and unanswered longer-term questions. Several women had just given up and had hysterectomies, which instead of eliminating problems as promised, just created a whole new set.

From my own point of view, it made no sense to put a young woman in a menopausal state to control or curtail gynaecological symptoms. I saw before me a life of continuously taking prescription medication to treat symptoms without ever getting to the root cause of the problem. That's when I began exploring complementary therapies and natural ways of dealing with my endometriosis.

A year or so after surgery, I started with acupuncture. At this time I was already experiencing a return of some of my old symptoms – a bit of rectal bleeding and some slight discomfort during my periods. Compared to my state before surgery, these really weren't worth mentioning, except that in the year since I'd realized just how much my lifestyle, relationships and sense of self had been affected by feeling so unwell for so long. I still had a lot of longer-term questions, but one thing I knew for sure was that I wanted to be as proactive as possible in managing my problems. I didn't want to mask or placate them again until they got so out of control that I was in constant pain and left with few options.

I also began looking for a new specialist. I wanted to work with an endocrinologist who was interested in treating me as a whole person and in exploring what exactly was happening. I wanted someone who was as interested in my quality of life as my reproductive chances, who could help me understand my body better, advise me on my choices and where necessary refer me to other specialists. I wanted someone who was also open to exploring complementary approaches.

After more time on the net, I found such a doctor and have been working with him for nearly three years. He has helped me to build up a network of specialists to maintain and improve my health including an acupuncturist, nutritionist, psychologist, physiotherapist and hormone specialist. All of these people, working together under my specialist's supervision, have proved to be an amazing combination.

When I first went to see my acupuncturist, I was taking birth control pills continuously for four months at a time as well as daily sinus medication, daily using an asthma inhaler, suffering from recurrent yeast infections and feeling generally run down. Within six months of seeing her, I had stopped taking any prescribed medication. She and my endocrinologist then began exploring the fundamental issues behind my ill health, including hormone imbalance, fungi and food intolerance, and worked together to help come up with the best treatment plan.

When my specialist diagnosed me with candida, he suggested I take antibiotics. I wanted to first check the possibility of a natural remedy with my acupuncturist, and he was completely open to this idea, adding that if I changed my mind we could try the antibiotics later. At another point I was experiencing some debilitating migraines. I went straight to my specialist, who gave me a prescription that provided much-needed temporary relief while he and my acupuncturist explored the possible causes. It's been the best of both worlds.

Four years after my surgery I take no prescription medicines, don't experience any major bowel issues, and have regular, essentially pain-free periods. At some point along the way it has become less about conquering my endometriosis and more about healing. My health is something I continue to need to monitor and address, but I've come to know my body very well and am able to intervene much faster and with a variety of approaches when something does arise, which keeps me in pretty good shape.

I am very grateful to all those who have helped me in the last four years to regain my health, including the surgeon. There is no doubt in my mind that without his knowledge and expertise I would not be where I am today. The surgery he performed gave me a starting point upon which all of the rest has been built.

Conventional Medicine

Strengths: Ability to prolong and save lives through new technology and scientific breakthroughs; treatment for acute conditions often very successful; advanced diagnostic and testing facilities; can deal with severe pain immediately and effectively; excellent for narrowing down possible reasons for symptoms.

Weaknesses: Pharmaceutical interference; prevention is not a part of the ethos, training or function; no form of nutrition training incorporated; doesn't look at the person holistically; compartmentalizes symptoms and refers accordingly, so you might find yourself being sent to two different specialists, when it is actually not necessary and just complicates things further; recommended treatment often masks symptoms instead of dealing with the root cause; tends to treat people only on the physical level.

Complementary Medicine

Strengths: Looks at the whole person – past and present; uses language more conducive to building new foundations that encourage patients to start an in-depth education about themselves and their health status; particularly good at linking together different, apparently unrelated, symptoms to find a common cause; works with nature, utilizing knowledge and awareness of the subtleties of how the body works, breaks down and heals; training can take many years, just as with orthodox medical training; a new breed of practitioners are enhancing their treatment by learning other necessary knowledge such as nutrition and muscle testing. Good at preventative work.

Weaknesses: Can overlook basic medical assessment; patient could have an acute condition (such as pneumonia) and be treated alternatively, which in such cases is inappropriate. Complementary medicine can provide support and treat many common maladies successfully. However, for serious conditions it is imperative that a GP or specialist is the primary assessor with the formal checks and tests in place. Whoever you choose to see can come across as being able to solve all your ills, but the body is complicated. Unless you are in a centre where different practitioners are striving for an integrated approach – with a central person asking the right questions and navigating you between your recommended lifestyle changes and towards the right therapy in the right order – your progress can be stilted and slow.

Be Organized

If you are at your wits' end because you are ill and have been to your GP or various complementary therapists, trying everything you can to get better – or if you have been told like Joanna and many others that you simply need to handle stress better, or that what you have doesn't exist – it is best to go back to basics. The reason it can seem frustrating and an upward climb at the beginning of anyone's journey has to do with a number of colliding factors, with a bit of mystery thrown in for good measure. You are probably dealing with a backlog of physiological baggage. The degree to which ailments have been suppressed or not dealt with – on top of any trauma, chaos, poor diet or lack of exercise – has to be dealt with first and foremost.

We have the huge advantage today of being able to learn a great deal about health problems and issues via the internet. It can educate and provide a basis for seeking help and further information. Knowing how overstretched GPs are, and how little time they have to spend with each patient, it can be very useful to do some research of your own before going to an appointment. Obviously, though, it's vital to use websites that offer reliable, accurate information.

I recommend Lynne McTaggart's What Doctors Don't Tell You, at www.wddty.co.uk. The site offers a searchable database on almost every illness, disease, condition and treatment option, both orthodox and complementary. Simply provide your search requirements and they will obtain and organize the information for you. Alternatively call 0870 444 9886.

You can also subscribe to the WDDTY newsletter, a publication that offers excellent advice and up-to-date information and opinions on all orthodox and complementary choices.

American medical specialist Dr Joseph Mercola also offers reliable, educational information at www.mercola.com

To make the most of the time you have with your GP or complementary practitioner, they need facts. In addition to your medical history, write down fully the relevant points about your symptoms. Knowing the key questions and recommendations will help you clarify what you need to address and understand your treatment options.

For a key questions checklist go to:
www.trifund.com/Data/healthathome/keyquest.htm

No Quick Fix

Due partly to the powerful marketing campaigns of the pharmaceutical industry and partly to our own laziness, a popular myth has evolved. We now believe that there is a pill to cure every ill. Therefore, we don't need to take care of ourselves – we'll just take a pill to make ourselves better. Many people go to their GPs expecting to come away with a prescription that will swiftly and efficiently take care of any problems without them having to change their lifestyle habits or address emotional stress. In reality, after a time the effects of most medications will wear off and can set off other reactions physiologically.

• Over the past decade, the number of antidepressant prescriptions in the UK has risen from under 10 million to more than 26 million each year.

Likewise, if you are continuously seeking to be fixed by one or more complementary therapies, followed by sabotaging yourself through a cocktail of poor eating, drink binging and/or drugs – you don't stand a chance of achieving your desired results. You will also end up putting an enormous strain on your whole system. Using the 'sticky plaster' mindset to rationalize self-sabotaging behaviour is a waste of everybody's time and your money. Instead, you should utilize complementary medicine intelligently through the stressful times, when you are feeling exhausted and below par, as well as using it to help prevent unwanted conditions naturally.

Antidepressants, non-steroid anti-inflammatory drugs, steroids, diet drugs, acne medication, Ritalin, anti-epilepsy drugs, anti-bacterial drugs, malaria tablets, puffers, blood-thinning drugs, beta blockers, the Pill and HRT all have a range of side effects. The degree to how these drugs are going to affect you can be horribly hit and miss. Some possible side effects of these prescription drugs are as follows: insomnia, excessive weight loss or gain, a breakdown of the auto-immune system, depression, intestinal and stomach bleeding, anorexia, sexual dysfunction, liver failure, nervous twitching/involuntary movements, heart palpitations, pulmonary hypertension, hallucinations, anxiety attacks, lowering of blood cell count, mood swings, skin conditions, constipation, headaches and more.

CASE STUDY – RITALIN

The history of Ritalin is just one example of the increasing number of nightmare cases of children and adults worldwide who have been prescribed medication for mental or physical disorders.

Ritalin is the best-known brand name for the drug methylphenidate and is prescribed for children diagnosed with Attention Deficit Hyperactivity Syndrome, or ADHD. This drug is an amphetamine and a stimulant. At its worst it has led to epileptic seizures and has been known to cause inflammation of the arteries of the brain. Other known side effects are psychosis, hallucinations, depression, obsessive compulsive behaviour, Tourette's syndrome, stunted growth and nausea, amongst others. Children taking this drug often appear to be in a zombie-like state – one effect of what is sometimes called 'chemical coshing'. There can also be a marked loss of appetite.

Ritalin was first marketed over 40 years ago, before drug companies were required to test for carcinogenicity. Toxicological tests were first completed in 1995, by which time millions of children had taken the drug. As a result of these tests, the manufacturer Novartis emphasizes that Ritalin should not be given to children under the age of six. Even so, the fact remains that in some countries the drug is being prescribed for children as young as two. Sales of this drug are continuing to soar – tripling worldwide in the last five years. The UK Department of Health says there are over 200,000 prescriptions processed each year, a hundredfold increase over the last decade. In America it is one of the most prescribed children's drugs with six million prescriptions a year and nearly $500 million in sales.

If your child is prescribed Ritalin, you do have other choices. Studies have shown that ADHD is often related to poor nutrition and that supplementation often significantly improves behaviour. Vitamin B6, magnesium, calcium, l-tryptophan and folic acid, alongside essential fatty acids, have a phenomenal impact in a high percentage of cases. Homeopathy has also been known to be extremely helpful, as have changes to environment and lighting (i.e. changing fluorescent lighting to daylight). Cranial-osteopathy has been used effectively coupled with either NLP or cognitive psychotherapy.

The Relationship Between Orthodox And Complementary Medicine

I have spent many years talking, working and researching extensively in all areas of orthodox and complementary medicine. And I have been told of and witnessed first-hand the arguments, breakthroughs and excitement surrounding new data, patients' recoveries, and other technological advances in both fields of medicine.

There is a myth that complementary therapies have no technology and that they consist only of promises, hocus-pocus, herbal potions and lotions. But, if the integration of complementary practices into the orthodox world is anything to go by, this perception couldn't be further from the truth.

The doctors and professors of medicine I've talked to have no problem in accepting that, in essence, orthodox medicine is not concerned with prevention. It is almost solely focused on disease – the pathology of it, the treating of it, and the research aspects of it. Diagnosis – learning how to recognize symptoms and what they mean – takes up 80 per cent of a student doctor's time.

Unfortunately, this emphasis on treatment rather than prevention places enormous power in the hands of the pharmaceutical industry, which makes the drugs and pills the medical profession prescribe. It's amazing how many professionals, orthodox and complementary alike, have complained to me about the extent to which the pharmaceutical industry has undermined the medical profession. I recently attended a talk on heart disease featuring one of England's leading heart specialists as well as a heart surgeon and a pharmacist who was also the managing director of his own company. I found both the specialist and surgeon fascinating and informative. The pharmacist, however, spent his part of the lecture giving us a blow-by-blow account of the profits he was going to rake in worldwide with new anti-cholesterol drugs he'd developed, boasting on top of that that he would be getting people as early as in their late twenties to start taking these drugs. When someone in the audience asked if it wouldn't be simpler if people just changed their diets, he answered: 'Why should they, when they can just take a pill?' Not once during the evening were preventative measures or changes in lifestyle, exercise or nutrition mentioned, let alone the long-term side effects. As an example, one of the most alarming (yet shockingly unknown) side effects of cholesterol-reducing drugs is the fact that they leech CoQ10, an essential nutrient found in the heart and brain, out of these organs. Clinical studies have definitively shown that reduced levels of Coq10 in the body puts additional strain on the heart as well as negatively affecting memory recall in the brain. Upon taking these drugs over an extended period of time, instances of Alzheimer's disease have also been seen to significantly increase.

• More than half of all British women have taken antidepressants at some point in their life.

Utilizing Medical And Complementary Training

Dr Shamim Daya trained as a GP and worked for the NHS for several years in the early 1990s. During this time she realized that seeing scores of patients a day for

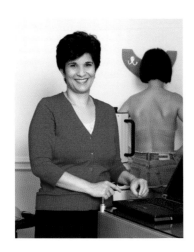

Dr Shamim Daya with the latest technology of Digital Infrared Thermal Imaging used for the early detection of breast abnormalities.

five minutes each and writing endless prescriptions was demoralizing both for her and her patients. Believing passionately that people should take better care of their own health, she started training in nutrition. At the same time, she experienced a personal health crisis. She was anemic and, looking back, had all of the symptoms of a weak thyroid. She was a strict vegetarian, but a very unhealthy one and didn't realize it. She was tired all the time, felt cold, her hair was falling out and her iron levels were very low. After successfully treating herself by improving her diet, she went on to make food therapy her specialty. In her private Harley Street practice, Shamim now incorporates kinesiology and Chinese medicine as well as thermal imaging, electrodermal testing and hair mineral analysis to check mineral and toxic metal status. She also uses urine tests to check hormonal status, as she finds these more accurate than blood tests. Alongside all of these she performs the standard blood tests and scans.

Shamim is an example of a new breed of highly trained medical practitioners incorporating in their work a truly thorough, all-round overview of all the factors that contribute to good health. As an example of her approach, she recounts the following case history. A young man suffering from depression came to see her for a second opinion after his GP recommended that he take antidepressants. When Shamim checked his nutritional status (as the GP, inevitably, had not) she found he was drinking eight cups of coffee with sugar each day, skipping breakfast, drinking half a bottle of wine every evening, and never drinking any water. On top of that he was running considerable distances three times per week. Being quite set in his ways, Shamim had to do a lot of work to persuade him just to drink water, change his eating habits and incorporate some stretching into his exercise regime. She explained that if he tried this for a week to see how it affected his depression, he could then make a comparison and, therefore, a more informed choice.

As she explained to me, this young man would almost certainly respond to antidepressants for the first three months and think, 'Great, they are working.' And yes, antidepressants are better than nothing. But typically what she sees with medication which merely masks symptoms is that the benefits are short-lived – after three months the drug doesn't work any more, or the patient needs higher doses. She says she knows this because she too once worked in this way. This is where the conventional medical system fails. The young man came back a week later and felt better. Slowly but surely over time, she persuaded him to make more changes, did the relevant tests, and within eight weeks he was perfectly well.

The role Shamim has taken on involves filling the gaps in the orthodox medical approach: checking her patients' diet, lifestyle and mineral status, and using Chinese medicine, particularly in checking the liver and the spleen. She says this is a language that orthodox doctors simply aren't taught, yet should be. She fully acknowledges that surgery is appropriate in many instances and medication can often work. Everything has its time and place. She feels that the only unfortunate thing is that when the medical system runs out of ideas and suggestions, they really don't know where to turn.

Shamim believes many doctors are beginning to question the existing system and are far more open-minded than they were even 10 years ago. As she points out, there are other practices besides hers where it is now common to see a doctor working alongside an osteopath, acupuncturist or homeopath.

The Power Of The Mind

Whether through stress, trauma, depression or a need for attention, the mind can be a major contributing factor where illness is concerned, hence why homeopathy is so adept in its prescription and its treatment. Homeopathy works through each person's emotional and mental constitution first and foremost (see also pages 80–81).

If you believe that something will or won't happen, then that will usually be the case. An individual's intention and will is very powerful, sometimes well beyond rational explanation. In 1960 for instance, a woman in Florida, US, called Mrs Maxwell Rogers, who weighed just 56kg, lifted the back of a 1,650kg car that had collapsed on her son when a jack slipped. She suffered multiple fractures in her spine in the effort, but saved her son's life.

If somebody chooses to believe that the combination of meditation, prayer and clean living is going to transform their situation, it often will. Obviously this is rare, but we have all seen, read or heard of stories where this has been the case. Equally, if somebody is adamant that changes to their food, lifestyle and treatment won't make any difference, there will be an even higher likelihood of a self-fulfilling prophecy. So, it really doesn't merit the energy debating the whys and wherefores of a positive result. There are so many people who are needlessly suffering or being extremely stubborn about looking outside their own little box. I have met a number of men who are taking medication for high cholesterol levels, blocked arteries and angina problems, but who refuse to address their nutrition or seek alternative input, and I find this both frustrating and depressing.

Several years ago, I was contacted by a very famous and well-respected man who looked like he was at death's door. He came to see me because his doctor had suggested that he do some very carefully supervised exercise. He was not overweight, but had cheated death medically for two or three decades. He'd undergone several heart bypass operations and was on a horrendous amount of medication. Discussing his nutrition, which was predictably diabolical, I had to conclude that he had made the decision a long time ago to have his cake and eat it too, regardless of the consequences. He had no intention of doing regular exercise or changing his diet – which he would have to do drastically but over a long period of time to be safe – nor of incorporating any complementary medicine to counter the toxicity of the drugs he was taking. He was a very nice man, we had a fair exchange that day and then he left. He died a couple of months later. He reminded me of my father, who had also lived a very socially active life, both personally and professionally, and who didn't want to seem less of a man by not partaking in the wines and foods all around him. He too died prematurely.

You Are In The Driver's Seat

The only person who can take control of your health is *you*. Your attitudes and belief systems, plus your knowledge or lack of it in this area, have a huge bearing on which direction you will choose to go. A heart specialist told me that when people experience a health scare, a good percentage – depending on age, generation, social class and predicament – visibly go in one of two directions. One group reacts by assuming that ill health is their route from now on – and doctors can almost see comfort, relief and expectancy in their demeanor as they accept the whole doctor, drug and hospital culture. Others get a real shock and desperately want to do whatever they can to get as far away as possible from a future filled with drugs, pills and operations. These two mindsets can be seen in individuals suffering from something as minor as a throat infection, through to gynaecological problems, male prostate issues, heart disease and cancer.

Autonomy And Health

One of the major benefits of not relying on drugs or misusing complementary medicine, while making the necessary changes in our nutrition and lifestyle, is autonomy.

However, remaining dependent on drugs both in the short and long term from babyhood upwards means big money for the drug companies. In a profit-driven world, can we really rely on the good-hearted kindness of the pharmaceutical industry to encourage individuals to look at how their unhealthy lifestyles result in ongoing physical symptoms, emotional distress and illness? Do we really expect them to encourage us to get our diet back in order and our sleep and exercise patterns on track? Of course not.

Drugs can, of course, be very useful initially in controlling acute conditions, and for pain relief. Yet, even here, there are few magic pills. Ninety per cent of drugs only work 30 per cent of the time, if that. Not to mention that each comes with a list of side effects in small print.

Let's take antibiotics for example. They have a powerful hold in people's belief systems. Of course, before penicillin was discovered, people died of many diseases such as pneumonia, tuberculosis, meningitis and blood poisoning. What is forgotten is that people also recovered from these diseases naturally and that for hundreds of years natural medicines derived from plants and herbs saved lives.

Antibiotics used thoughtlessly and excessively affect everyone's well-being. They make us vulnerable to bacteria, which mutate and become resistant to drugs. They reduce our own inbuilt mechanisms for fighting infections. They strip our gut of bacteria, good and bad, and allow fungal infections such as candida to flourish and become systemic. They can cause side effects such as skin disorders, liver and kidney dysfunction and heart palpitations. These side effects are always described as rare, though, because no one fills out the yellow card – on which all suspected reactions to new and established medicines are recorded – any more. Often patients don't associate their nausea and itchy skin with the course of antibiotics they've just taken. Yet I have seen more people suffering candida than practically any other problem bar weight issues. If we are not given drugs to clear out the candida, we resort to buying topical medicatal creams over the counter. From an energetic perspective, antibiotics divert the vital force, our internal energy, from the job at hand. They suppress the action of all energetic work in the body, and physically suppress the action and reason for the infection in individuals. They set people back in time in their individual journey towards health, meaning the problem will almost inevitably recur or result in unwanted side effects.

There are thousands of deaths and adverse reactions every year due to prescription drugs. Clearly, taking them can all too easily just create a new set of problems. So take the power back into your own hands. Let your GP and complementary practitioners know that you are open to their advice, but make it clear that you are unwilling to take medication endlessly as a solution to a health problem. Then, when you really need to take antibiotics for an acute or life-threatening situation, they have the maximum chance of being effective.

Concept Of Holism

There are many ways to explain the concept of holism, which looks at the whole rather than individual processes. Consider the factors that could be maintaining back pain for instance. Postural discrepancies, work pressures, computer use, emotional worries, family stresses, not exercising or exercising incorrectly, seating, your bed, structural anatomical problems and so on.

Each person's canvas is a vast and complex one. If the right questions are asked so that the advice given to you can be prioritized – starting by locating the causes followed by what changes you can make yourself in every area, later adding in the right complementary help – there will be a big difference in the outcome and your ability to maintain good health.

Getting and staying well is very similar to learning a new language. First you learn the basic words you need to get by, then you learn the structure and the grammar, then you build your vocabulary until finally you are able to put it all together. Learning to drive is much the same. At first it seems impossible, but you go through your process of trial and error and before you know it, it becomes second nature and you have it for life.

The Five 'Bodies' Of The Human Being

As we evolve and as new strains of bugs, viruses and illnesses show themselves, both orthodox and complementary medical systems strive to keep up. The medical fraternity acknowledges that disease can exist on a physical and mental level – the basis for current medical and psychological practices. Complementary medicine in its varied formats accepts that disease can exist as a result of physical and mental/emotional trauma. However, as a new breed of integrated doctors and practitioners strives to bridge the gap between orthodox and complementary medicine, a new paradigm is emerging. One of the biggest influences in establishing this new inclusive medical model is neurologist Dr Dietrich Klinghardt, who has developed a system called 'The Five Levels of Healing', as well as a highly reliable method of bio-energetic testing called Autonomic Response Testing, or ART.

Since 1988, Dr Klinghardt has been an influential speaker, teacher and workshop leader at numerous medical conferences worldwide. In recent years, he has also emerged as one of the leading voices on the issues of heavy metal and environmental toxicity. His detoxification method, using a combination of plants, Qigong (Chinese energy balancing) and energy psychology techniques, has found widespread acceptance in several European countries and in the US.

Led by Dr Klinghardt, eminent neurological surgeons, doctors and dentists, as well as many complementary practitioners, are integrating and utilizing these techniques. His system has been constructed in such a way that it is now available to both orthodox and complementary practitioners from any philosophy or belief system, who wish to approach an individual's needs from the highest possible level of integrity and accuracy. His understanding of human beings as more than just their physical bodies, combined with the precise methods of direct resonance testing now being developed, provide a ground-breaking explanation for one of the most persistent medical mysteries – why one remedy works for one person and not for another.

We are beginning to understand that hereditary factors, chemicals and other pollutants, nutrition, exercise and lifestyle choices can play a significant role in the creation or manifestation of disease. We are also becoming more aware of how the choices our mother made while she was carrying us can affect us later in life. For example, many of you are aware that if a pregnant woman smokes cannabis or cigarettes or drinks too much alcohol, it will directly affect the developing embryo. But this also extends to whether your mother ate poorly or simply had unresolved emotional problems while pregnant. All these factors can have an impact on your immune system health and well-being, your susceptibility to disease and your ability to recover throughout your life. New methods of testing through direct energy resonance are able not only to detect precisely these influences, but also enable the practitioner to resolve them, utilizing a highly individualized approach.

At the heart of Dr Klinghardt's research and work is his conclusion that we all have five 'bodies' that can influence our health. They are the physical body, the electromagnetic body (feelings), the mental body (attitudes/beliefs), the intuitive body (symbols/dreams/meditative states) and the spiritual body (oneness with God, or however you perceive or experience this).

Let me give you an example. Consider the following: Why do some people, who are exposed to mercury, for example, deposit the toxin in their hypothalamus (and develop multiple hormone problems), others in the limbic system (depression), others in the adrenals (fatigue), some in the long bones (osteoporosis, leukemia), some in the pelvis (interstitial cystitis), others in the autonomic and sensory ganglia (chronic pain syndromes), some in the connective tissue (scleroderma, lupus), some in the cranial nerves (tinnitus, cataracts, loss of sense of smell) and others in the muscles (fibromyalgia)? Multiple reasons can be identified, including:

Past physical trauma: Traumas such as a closed head injury, a backwards or upwards blow to any part of the skull or face, whiplash, or a vigorous tooth extraction will make the brain susceptible to becoming a storage site for heavy metals including lead, aluminum and mercury.

Food allergies: These often cause a low-grade encephalitis or joint inflammation. Again, this makes these areas more likely to become targets for toxic deposits.

Geopathic and electromagnetic stress: A significant number of people sleeping on underground water lines or too close to electrical equipment are experiencing adverse health reactions.

Scars and teeth: Both of these can create abnormal electrical signals, which then alter the function of the autonomic nervous system.

Environmental toxins: Solvents, pesticides and wood preservatives have a synergistic effect with most toxic metals. Metals will often accumulate in body parts that have been chemically injured at a prior time.

Unresolved trauma: Unresolved psycho-emotional trauma or problems in the family system can affect the physical body in many ways.

TMJ/Occlusion: The health of the jaw joint can affect our general heath (see also page 68).

This may sound complicated, but it really isn't. In practice, the five 'bodies' and the factors that can influence each body can be reliably tested and treated using both orthodox and complementary approaches.

Autonomic Response Testing

Autonomic Response Testing or ART enables practitioners to diagnose in a holistic yet scientific and reliable way, recognizing disorders of the physical, emotional, mental and intuitive bodies – four of the five levels of healing identified by Dr Klinghardt.

A major part of this work involves finding and treating the root cause of the symptoms one is experiencing, which is often the most overlooked obstacle to healing. Known as interference fields, the root cause may be a scar, a damaged tooth, an old injury or an unresolved emotional issue. Working with the autonomic nervous system, practitioners are able to locate and treat this root cause of trauma, pain or discomfort. In many cases, such pain or trauma has either been long forgotten or suppressed, but by accessing the issue via the unconscious mind, the problem can be resolved – often permanently.

By using ART, it is possible to accurately determine the most appropriate course of treatment. On the physical level it could be a herb, vitamin or mineral which resolves symptoms that originate from either ingesting or being in contact with solvents or heavy metal toxins, major food allergies, chemical sensitivities (toothpaste included), or other allergic problems in the body. On an emotional or mental level, ART can direct us via colour therapy or tapping on certain access points on the body, known as energy meridians, to resolve painful issues that are not allowing the body to heal.

ART uses muscle testing to determine the state of the person. Each of the four tested levels or 'bodies' of the person can be highly functional or to a varying degree dysfunctional. Through this medium the body will deal with issues in order of priority. The most urgent problems show up first; the less acute later. This may continue until all major issues are resolved.

This form of testing can be very thorough and comprehensive. And because it views the body as one cohesive unit with no part isolated from another, it can be used in a variety of orthodox and complementary settings. I know of two dentists in the UK who have found that using ART has transformed how they work and has, without a doubt, elevated the quality and efficiency of their treatments.

Dentistry Combined With ART

Dr Marina Carew feels that it is unfortunate that medical and dental professionals have not fully recognized the connection between the health of the mouth and illnesses, even though a link has been established between patients with chronic gum disease and heart disease, strokes, premature births and still-births. Dr Reinhard Voll, a renowned German physician, concluded after more than 40 years of research and observation that almost 80 per cent of illness is related entirely or partially to problems in the mouth. I have heard this incredible statistic more than once from various practitioners.

ART posits a list of seven factors that stress the body, leading to what Dr Klinghardt calls 'blocked regulation'. Three of these can be related to the mouth.

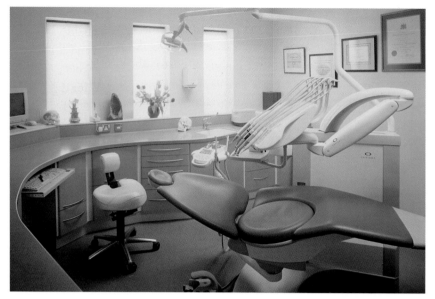

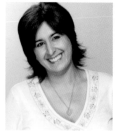

Dr Marina Carew is one of the new breed practising Holistic Integrated Dentistry which incorporates the knowledge of conventional dentistry with Eastern and Western medicine.

Heavy-metal toxicity results from mercury in amalgams; palladium and nickel in crowns and bridges; cobalt chrome in dentures; and cadmium in root canal fillings. The vast majority of people, including many physicians, do not realize that the silver fillings in their tooth cavities can consist of up to 50 per cent mercury, an extremely toxic substance.

Mercury as elemental vapour is found in dental amalgams and in trace amounts in the air, while traces of inorganic mercury compounds are found in the air as well as water and many foods. Organic mercury (methyl mercury) is present in trace amounts in the air, as well as in fish, especially predatory species such as tuna, shark and swordfish.

Dr Carew was taught at dental school that the mercury in dental amalgams was 'locked in' and therefore harmless, but scientific evidence now suggests that mercury vapour escapes from silver fillings continuously, and, indeed, that the rate of release increases immediately after chewing and brushing. Heat also increases the rate of release of mercury vapour. World Health Organization (WHO) studies in 1992 concluded that the greatest body burden of mercury was from the vapour released from dental amalgam fillings. The WHO also stated that there is no safe minimum dose of mercury.

Corrosion of amalgam in the mouth is a problem that arises because amalgam contains four or five different metals. When the saliva, acting as an electrolyte (or conductor), mixes these different metals, it produces a battery effect which increases the amount of mercury vapour released and also results in the creation of a small measurable electric current. This phenomenon is known as 'oral galvanism'.

When other metals such as gold are placed in a mouth containing amalgam, mercury release may be increased tenfold.

TMJ/Occlusion: The health of the jaw joint, the temporomandibular joint or TMJ, and the way the teeth bite together (occlusion) are very important to good health. Three major energy meridians – relating to the endocrine system, the stomach and the large intestine – intersect at the site of the TMJ. The lower jaw, the mandible, is connected to the skull at the TM joints. When the disc is slightly displaced or the condyle is positioned too far backwards and upwards, clicks or pops may be heard on opening, closing or chewing. This may be a sign of joint dysfunction, or TMD. TMD can be the result of trauma such as a blow to the head or face, whiplash injuries, an occlusion (bite) problem, or poor development of the jaws.

Symptoms of TMD may include one or more of the following: headaches, migraines, neck pain, shoulder pain, lower back pain, palpitations, fatigue, clenching and/or grinding of the teeth, tinnitus, blocked ears, stuffy ears, loss of hearing, sore throat, swollen lymph glands, vertigo, itchy ears, sensation of something stuck in the throat, poor posture, sinusitis or stomach problems.

A simple test to determine whether someone may be suffering from TMD is to try to insert the middle three fingers into the fully open mouth so that the index finger is against the upper teeth and the ring finger is touching the lower teeth. If this is not possible, then the opening is restricted and further investigation should be undertaken.

Interference fields from scars or teeth can put the body under a great deal of stress. A dead tooth, a cavity or gum disease can be a focus of infection. What's more, the infection produced may target specific organs.

In addition to being a physician, Dr Reinhard Voll was also a professor of anatomy and an acupuncturist. During his 40 years of research, he identified a network of energetic pathways which he believed ran throughout the body. Many of these correspond to the Chinese acupuncture meridians, but there are also many new pathways. These pathways connect each tooth with specific organs, vertebrae, joints, tissue systems and endocrine glands. A patient may have, for example, a heart condition which Dr Voll's system would identify as resulting from a wisdom tooth infection. Equally, a problem in an organ may cause the death of a tooth along the same acupuncture meridian. For instance, a bladder problem could lead to a dead incisor.

Using ART or electro-acupuncture as devised by Dr Voll, a dentist is able to determine if an energy blockage in a tooth or cavity is causing problems elsewhere in the body along the same meridian, or vice versa.

Holistic Integrated Dentistry

Dr Evelien van Amerongen also uses ART in her dental practice. Evelien has been a practicing dentist since 1981. From the beginning, she has been interested in merging conventional dental practices with complementary approaches. Today her Holistic Integrated Dentistry practice in London provides one of the most comprehensive approaches to dentistry in the UK.

Evelien finds that setting aside the popularity of a 'pretty smile', most people choose to ignore the importance of their teeth. Comments like 'I hate the dentist' have their origin in the 'drill 'em, fill 'em, whack 'em and pack 'em' practices fuelled by images of dentists pinning their patients to the chair in order to carry out their procedures. These negative images are reflected in the high proportion of phobic patients. Astonishingly, 60 per cent of the UK population seldom or never visit the dentist, except in emergencies. Of the remaining 40 per cent, only one in five attend on a regular, six-monthly basis. Misconceptions, misinformation and past approaches have resulted in national dental awareness being left far behind in the twenty-first century.

Holistic Integrated Dentistry (HID) incorporates the knowledge of conventional dentistry with Eastern and Western medicine. Initial health assessments on a 'whole being' basis address symptoms, causality and prevention in ways which go far beyond the tooth structure itself.

The teeth have an energetic relationship with the rest of the body on a biochemical, structural, sensory, emotional and electromagnetic level; therefore, the state of our teeth has a huge impact on our overall health. Someone's general health is clearly depicted by the state of their teeth and oral environment, and by using dental intervention alongside general health care, improvements are often quite dramatic. Issues targeted include fear and phobic behaviour, diet, saliva ph, mercury fillings, battery effect, extraction sites, root canal treatment, jaw/bite alignment, gum disease, infections and lumps and bumps.

The Toxicity Of Fillings

The toxic mercury vapour released by chewing on mercury and amalgam fillings mixes with food, entering our digestive system and adding to the body's burden of heavy metals. As a fat-loving substance, mercury has a strong affinity to fatty tissues such as the brain, liver, kidneys and the cell wall. Incorporated into all cell membranes, mercury affects each cell's capacity to detoxify itself, inevitably causing premature cell death. Once the liver and gall bladder are affected by mercury, the body loses its capacity to clean and rid itself of its toxins and heavy metals, leading to a vicious circle of intoxication. To rectify this problem, the source of mercury has to be removed and underlying infections recognized.

In dentistry, the removal of toxic fillings has become increasingly popular, both for cosmetic and health reasons. But it is vital that it is done with care and skill. Both Dr Carew and Dr van Amerongen make the point that removal of mercury amalgam fillings without proper health assessments and protective protocols only adds to the body's burden of heavy metals. Appropriate time needs to be taken to prepare the body, using nutritional and whole food supplementation to boost elimination routes (via stools, urine, sweat or breath) for the toxins. Once the body releases the mercury, underlying viruses, parasites and bacteria are exposed to the body's immune system. It is therefore important to have the right nutritional, pharmaceutical and homeopathic medicines available to help the body deal with the effects of any infection.

There are several ways to safely remove amalgam and it is imperative to find a dentist who follows one of them. It may also be very dangerous to have several amalgams removed over a short space of time.

Marina Carew's recommendations include pre-operative nutritional advice to ensure that the bowel is functioning properly as it is the main excretory organ for mercury; supplements if it is necessary to build up the immune system; a well-ventilated surgery; protective clothing and glasses; and a post-operative detoxification programme.

Dr Klinghardt has his own protocol using chlorella, fish oils, freeze-dried garlic, coriander and selectrolytes, amongst other supplements, which Evelien van Amerongen has also found to be very effective. ART can be used to determine which supplements are needed for the detoxification process for each individual patient.

Due to mercury's complex symptomology and fat-soluble nature, conventional blood tests, stool and urine testing cannot actually reveal the real body burden of heavy metals. ART however allows doctors, dentists and complementary practitioners to identify which heavy metal is stored where in the body, enabling them to target a specific organ for the appropriate detoxification and nutritional/medicinal support. This can include acupuncture, homeopathy, light frequency therapy, chiropractic, cranial-sacral therapy, oxidation and ozone therapy.

For more information see www.greatsmile.org.uk

Lilias Curtin, an Autonomic Response Testing and Electronic Gem Therapy practitioner.

Complementary Therapies Combined With ART

Lilias Curtin is emerging as one of the UK's leading ART practitioners. A

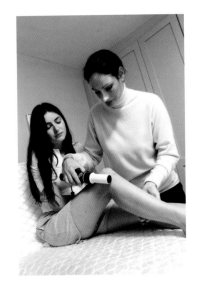

complementary practitioner in London since 1999, Lilias was one of the first accredited Magnet Therapists in the UK and is also trained in Electronic Gem Therapy. Lilias has found that Autonomic Response Testing allows her to expand her testing and understanding of what is happening within each person's body, which enables her to be even more specific with the other therapies she offers.

By using ART, Lilias is able to tailor a treatment to an individual's unique body, energy and circumstances. She is well-known for being at the cutting edge of energy medicine and is always exploring new ways of treating people. She continually pushes the boundaries that exist in many treatments to see if there are better ways to progress. Using ART, Lilias is able to test whether an individual requires colour treatment, Electronic Gem Therapy, a remedy or supplement, Mental Field Therapy, Aqua Detox or Magnet Therapy.

Only through comprehensively testing and listening to each person's many levels can the best method of treatment be revealed.

CASE STUDY – M'S STORY

M is a 57-year-old woman who consulted Lilias in 2003. She was aware that a lot was going wrong in her life, but had been unable to find the right answers, or even be sure what questions she should be asking. M was depressed, overweight, had little energy, was suffering from the shock of a car accident, had been diagnosed previously with helicobacter and thought she may also have parasites.

On her first visit, M was found through ART to have mercury toxicity and candida, as suspected. Her intestines were very tender, so she was treated with Electronic Gem Therapy which seemed to make her a lot more comfortable. She left with mercury detox protocols to follow and a supplement to combat the candida. On her second visit, she stated that she felt brighter and that her energy levels had improved. She was now ready to face some of the root causes of her discomfort. By using ART combined with Mental Field Therapy, she was able to deal with long-standing personal issues related to her marriage, which were manifesting themselves as intestinal problems.

On M's third visit she was much more positive in her outlook and behaviour. Using ART, four different types of parasites were discovered in her system, which accounted for the fact that she permanently felt bloated and large around the middle. Three types of fungi were also found. Food testing was conducted to see what foods her body could not tolerate due to the parasites and fungi, and it was recommended that she avoid these foods for approximately six weeks while her body eliminated the parasites and the fungi.

Two appointments later M was alert, vibrant and sassy. She had gone from a size 16 to a size 12 and lost inches around her waist. Friends could not stop commenting about her new look and she felt good about herself. She was able to talk more freely about some of the issues that had always haunted her. On testing her, the parasites were found to have been completely eradicated although there was still a small trace of the fungi.

Over the course of seven appointments, M improved physically, emotionally and psychologically. Most foods were re-introduced back into her diet and she is virtually clear of the fungi. Her demeanour has totally changed for the better and her relationship with her husband is much improved.

Tapping For Health

Emotional Freedom Technique (EFT) and Mental Field Therapy (MFT) have evolved from Thought Field Therapy (TFT), a unique method of healing developed by American psychotherapist Dr Roger Callahan. These methods involve tapping on the body's energy meridians to bring about powerful emotional and physical healing. Grief, anger, phobias, post-traumatic stress disorders, guilt, headaches, pain and asthma can be dramatically, easily and quickly relieved using these healing tapping techniques. Tapping can also be employed to improve skills such as public speaking or to ease examination nerves.

Electronic Gem Therapy uses the properties of precious gemstones to induce energy into diseased or injured tissue, organs and glands.

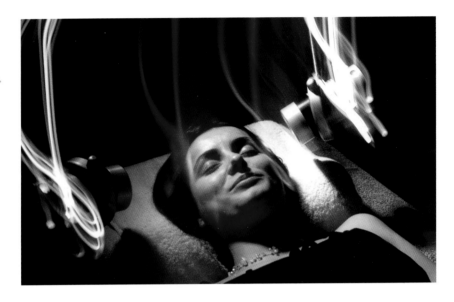

• 95 per cent of people with eczema rely on using steroid-based creams.

Electronic Gem Therapy

Electronic Gem Therapy or EGT, which should not be confused with crystal, colour or modern light therapy, uses the properties of precious gemstones to induce energy into diseased or injured tissue, organs and glands via sympathetic resonance. Many infections, allergies, psychological and physical illnesses cause an imbalance in the organs and glands. Gem Therapy is able to correct these imbalances by adjusting the biological activity of organs and energy imbalances. Today, surgical laser beams are generated by rubies, but many precious gemstones have been valued for their healing properties for thousands of years. Some Tibetan and Indian medicines are made from the fine powder of gemstones.

Gemstones are reservoirs of pure radiating energy and the colour of a gemstone determines its effect on living cells. Gemstone rays pass through the body and influence cellular behaviour in a similar way to infrared rays. The concentrated rays of gemstones influence cellular activity at an atomic level, where gross chemicals such as herbs and drugs cannot penetrate.

For example, some diseases such as burns, sprains, new injuries and pain are all areas of high temperature and excessive energy emission, requiring a cooling and calming gemstone treatment. Conversely, other forms of illness such as allergies, asthma and old injuries are characterized by low temperature and low energy emissions. These invariably benefit from stimulating and invigorating gemstone energy. With EGT it is possible to energize one part of the body, while at the same time soothing another.

Electronic Gem Therapy (which can be used with ART) is a complete therapy in itself, proving to be particularly successful in treating adults and children with eczema and asthma.

Here is one little boy's story.

CASE STUDY – AIDEN'S STORY

Lilias first met three-year-old Aiden and his parents in April 2002. Aiden had been suffering from severe eczema since he was four months old. Searching for some much-needed relief, the family travelled from Newcastle to London to try Electronic Gem Therapy.

Quite often, particularly through the winter months, 90 per cent of Aiden's body would be covered in eczema. His face would become especially raw and encrusted from itching and infection. This would then spread over his scalp.

Aiden's parents had to wrap his body in paste bandages to cover the raw, itching skin, trying to prevent scarring and infection. Because of Aiden's age he could not control the desire to scratch, and if left unattended for even a few minutes, this would result in cracked and bleeding skin. This meant that one parent had to be by his side keeping a vigilant lookout at all times.

The many sleepless nights and Aiden's constant discomfort had taken its toll on the entire family. Everyone was exhausted. His parents were also beginning to fear that if the eczema continued at its present level, then Aiden would not be able to attend school regularly as the demands of looking after him would simply be too great – not to mention the eczema's stigmatizing effect. Having tried all the traditional treatments of cortisone creams and steroid injections, as well as a few alternative treatments, with no success, the parents regarded Electronic Gem Therapy as a last resort.

At Aiden's first consultation, Lilias observed that his body was extremely hot and irritated. As is often the case with eczema, the liver appeared to be overactive, while the spleen appeared underactive. The first priority was to bring these two organs into balance. Lilias was able to calm the liver by using gem lamps filled with emeralds and sapphires. At the same time she was able to activate the spleen and improve blood quality by using lamps filled with diamonds and carnelians. Lastly, she directed a gem lamp of sapphires towards the crown of the head for an overall emotionally balancing effect.

When Aiden returned for his second appointment just one week later, his skin was showing visible improvement. The body was cooler and the eczema patches generally smaller. At Aiden's third appointment, the eczema patches were even smaller and his parents reported that he seemed to be much less itchy, particularly on his back. Overall, his skin was looking much better – clearer, smoother and less irritated. As the itching decreased, Aiden was able to sleep better and he was showing signs of improved energy and demeanour as well.

After just five weeks and four treatments, the patches of eczema around Aiden's head and neck were significantly reduced and the itching was continuing to subside. Overall his parents reported that he was scratching less, sleeping better and appeared calmer. In addition, a significant milestone had been reached. For the first time in his life, Aiden's parents were able to leave him for short periods without supervision.

Aiden saw Lilias for three more treatments over the next few months, and after each treatment his eczema continued

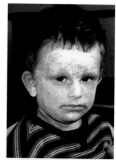
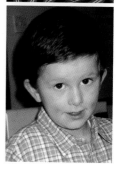

(Above) Aiden, who suffered from very bad eczema, before and after 7 sessions of Electronic Gem Therapy with Lilias Curtin. (Below) A sample of various precious gemstones used for Electronic Gem Therapy.

to subside until it disappeared. After years of doctors' appointments, medication and bandages, Aiden's eczema was successfully treated with Electronic Gem Therapy in just seven appointments between April and November 2002.

In 2004, two years after Aiden's Electronic Gem Therapy treatments, his parents report that he has remained eczema-free. He is living the life of a healthy five-year-old, no longer misses out on activities with friends or siblings, and has successfully started school.

Native American Healing

Dr Mary Hoptroff believes that each person is his or her own greatest healer. A GP for the past 20 years, she is also a highly qualified holistic healer who specializes in the Native American art of energetic medicine, based on the ancient medicine wheel. This wheel has eight points, as in a compass. An 'upset' in one of these points, such as an unresolved or difficult experience, manifests itself as disease – physical, emotional, intellectual or energetic. Conversely, disease itself can cause an 'upset'. Either way, Mary believes that understanding any imbalance in a person's medicine wheel is the first stage of healing. Her integrated approach to energetic and orthodox diagnosis is highly unusual and effective.

Mary further believes that every body has a core energy comprising 10 points that rise from the abdomen, travelling up the spine to above the head. Each point connects to the body physically or emotionally, mentally or energetically. When each point is functioning, all is well. When one or more points are lacking or over-energized, an imbalance occurs. And this results in disease.

Understanding these 10 energy points is the key to complete health. People can learn how to access their energy points, renew them and protect them against being drained. As they learn this, Mary also helps her patients to focus on specific goals throughout the process so that they can begin to tap into energy sources they didn't know they had.

Holistic Physiotherapy

Jacqueline Flexney-Briscoe is one of the few physiotherapists in Britain combining connective tissue manipulation, manual lymph drainage, the MacKenzie technique and cranial-sacral therapy in private practice. Over the past four years, she has successfully treated over 1,000 patients with spinal problems and a further 1,300 with other musculo-skeletal problems. Like all the doctors and practitioners mentioned here, Jacqueline firmly believes that you cannot treat any part of the body in isolation. She describes connective tissue as being like a spider's web that goes around every muscle and every joint, through the skin, around the stomach and around the blood vessels – everywhere through the body, with an overlap of connective tissue from one area to another.

As we get older, our bodies tighten up. We are no longer able to suck on our big toe as we could as a baby. Mental and emotional stresses and strains from work, family and life in general get taken on board as an increase in physical tension.

• Four out of five British GPs overprescribe Prozac and similar drugs to people suffering from depression or anxiety.

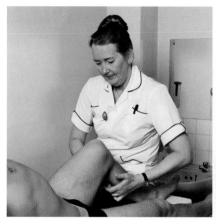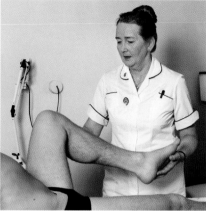

Jacqueline Flexney-
Briscoe is one of the few
physiotherapists in Britain
combining connective
tissue manipulation,
manual lymph drainage,
the MacKenzie technique
and cranio-sacral therapy
in private practice.

These tense areas of the body (often backs, necks and joints such as ankles and elbows) then become vulnerable to injury. For example, many of Jacqueline's back patients have just moved house. They have all of the stress that comes with moving house, then just before or just after the move they do something physical and their back suffers the consequences. Had they done the same physical activity at any other time, it probably wouldn't have been a problem. It is the same with many of the physical injuries that she sees. The timing of the injury has a stress-related element.

If you take the tension out of the spider's web, out of the connective tissue, the body becomes more forgiving, more elastic and allows for more flexibility physically, mentally and emotionally.

CASE STUDY – B'S STORY

Jacqueline tells of a man, B, who came to her with a sport-related ankle injury. As the chief accountant for a building society, this man carried huge responsibility. Jacqueline treated his Achilles tendon problem with connective tissue manipulation. Returning for a follow-up appointment, he asked if this treatment could possibly be helping his indigestion. Apparently, he had been experiencing awful indigestion every Monday morning and every Monday lunchtime for a year. He was terribly crotchety and always had to take a three-week holiday because it took him one week to relax, one week to enjoy himself, and one week to build up to going back to work. At the weekend, his children wouldn't approach him before lunch on Saturday because he was so wound up, and Sunday nights were no good either because he was getting ready to go back to work. His family therefore did very little at the weekend because of his stressful state.

When Jacqueline finished treating his ankle, he asked if she would carry on treating his indigestion, which she did, and it disappeared completely. As this happened, he was getting generally less and less stressed, and, when presented with new challenges at work, he could cope with them quite happily. Before, his mindset had been: 'What if I make a mistake, what am I going to do, will I be able to handle things if something goes

wrong?' Weekends are now normal and active, and no one has to tiptoe round him.
Holidays can now be a long weekend or more.

Reiki

Reiki is a system of energy healing that is simple yet has far-reaching effects. It is thought to have its roots in ancient Buddhism and was introduced to the West from Japan in the late 1930s. There are no religious connotations within Reiki, and no belief system is necessary to practise or receive this method of healing. Central to Reiki is the concept that we are energetic beings, who are made up of and surrounded by energy. The energy flow within us supports life by helping to maintain homeostasis, or balance, between body, mind and spirit. This energy is known as Ki. When Ki is diminished ill health can arise.

The main aim of Reiki is to bring about balance and harmony in mind, body and spirit, increasing one's sense of well-being. In keeping with Eastern thought, this balance and harmony combined with free-flowing energy (Ki) are all vital to our well-being. A professional Reiki practitioner should not impose their own spiritual belief system on to the client nor should they claim to be doing the healing. The practitioner is merely the channel that the energy flows through.

It is important to note that anyone with serious medical problems should always be seen by a doctor prior to receiving Reiki. Another important point to consider is that the word 'healing' means many things to many people. A Reiki practitioner should not talk in terms of curing disease, but rather emphasize that Reiki will potentially help support the body on many levels.

Studies have shown that Reiki induces a relaxation effect which has been monitored by changes in breathing rate, pulse rate and blood pressure. Given that science now recognizes the link between stress and illness, Reiki can be used as a tool for relaxation and stress relief. Anecdotal evidence from practitioners and recipients suggests that the effects of Reiki go beyond relaxation. This is a skill that is incredibly simple to use, and anybody can do it. Reiki can help you sleep, recover from an illness or operations, or relax you, your partner, friends and children at any time.

Carole practising Reiki on a client's teenage daughter, who finds it reduces stress and anxiety during exams, for example.

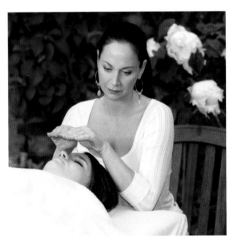

Many parents I know and their children have done an initial two-day Reiki course. It gives the children a great sense of responsibility and teaches them how to help themselves in times of trouble and illness. This is a very inexpensive, all-purpose tool to have available.

I have also found that often on arrival at a class a client may be suffering from stomach pains, a headache, is upset or simply exhausted. As a result I will spend 10 or 15 minutes Reiki-ing them, and it always makes a substantial difference to how they feel.

Liz Hawkins, a Reiki master, believes that Reiki works on the physical, emotional and spiritual levels to bring about a return to wholeness. She originally began her career over 20 years ago as a registered nurse; however, like so many others she realized that orthodox medicine did not hold all the answers. This led her on a path of learning toward a more holistic approach incorporating massage, aromatherapy, reflexology and Reiki.

Liz's belief that orthodox and complementary medicine could work together led her to develop therapies for a cancer centre which included offering Reiki during orthodox cancer treatment. The uptake by patients is impressive, feedback is very positive, and most patients report feeling an increased sense of calm and peace following a session. Other reported benefits include less pain and fear and more energy. Often a patient will say that the Reiki got them through a difficult treatment for a serious condition.

Healing And The NHS

Healing – often known as spiritual healing or therapeutic touch – is a skill with a recorded history of over four thousand years. Misunderstood and underused, healing is a natural phenomenon that is profoundly relaxing, restorative and completely non-invasive. It can be of therapeutic value for a wide range of physical and psychological conditions, sometimes to a remarkable degree, and it can be employed by itself or in conjunction with any other therapy.

Healing involves a transfer of energy between the healer and the patient to deal with stress, aid the patient's immune system and promote self-healing mechanisms. Healers concentrate on the patient with focused intent, either panning the hands at varying distances above the surface of the body or sometimes using light touch. The resulting interaction of energy enables the depleted energy of the patient to benefit from the energy radiated by or through the healer. The process does not require either the patient or the practitioner to be religious.

The Doctor-Healer Network (DHN) was founded in the UK in 1988 by a group of doctors who were working with healers, its prime aim being to encourage the promotion of healing within the NHS. Today, there are an increasing number of healers working in NHS environments.

According to the DHN, healing is a powerful natural relaxant and restorative. It is proven scientifically to bring about a beneficial effect on stressed or damaged enzymes, seeds, plants and animals and to accelerate the healing of simple injuries in humans. In a review of over 150 controlled studies of healing, the DHN points out that more than half demonstrated significant effects.

While the Network has tended to focus on expanding their work in Primary Care Trusts, there have also been some quite significant breakthroughs within hospitals. Angie Buxton, one of London's DHN members, heads a team of complementary therapists including healers at University College and Middlesex hospitals, attached to the haematology departments. Angie says that medical and nursing staff have been so impressed by the beneficial effects of healing and other complementary therapies, particularly in terms of patients' quality of life, that NHS funding has been acquired to support her team's work. Annie Hallet, a nurse and healer, is doing similar work in hospitals in East Anglia. A number of DHN members have also established links with local general practices, and now provide healing sessions within these practices.

All healers who are members of the DHN subscribe to a recognised code of conduct, carry professional indemnity insurance and have undertaken a recognized course of training. Many GPs are trained healers as well.

For more information, contact the Doctor-Healer Network, 27 Montefiore Court, Stamford Hill, London N16 5TY; tel/fax: 020 8800 3569.

Act Before You Reach Crisis Point

Dr Rosy Daniel has witnessed over and over again how too many people wait for an immense crisis such as a cancer diagnosis to act as a wake-up call. Only then do they seem able to find the energy and motivation to change poor eating, sleeping and exercise habits, negative ways of thinking and destructive behavioural patterns.

Rosy's mission is to help people who are not yet ill make life-affirming, positive health changes – before they are frightened to death by a crisis into taking action. Working as an Integrated Medicine Consultant at the Harley Street Cancer Centre in London and in Bristol, she has devised her highly innovative Health Creation Programme. Over a six-month period, Health Creation mentors help individuals, teams or organizations shift their ethos – personally and collectively – to one of respect and a nurturing relationship with themselves, other people and the environment.

Formerly Medical Director and CEO of the world-famous Bristol Cancer Help Centre, Rosy studied shiatsu, yoga, meditation and transpersonal psychology as well as conventional medicine. She says that once she started work in the Bristol Centre, everything she had intuitively felt about the link between mind and body was confirmed as she witnessed truly remarkable recoveries from cancer. People, she says, became well from the inside out.

- One in three people will be affected by cancer.

Initially, she was deeply in awe of the doctors, healers and therapists at the Bristol Centre. They seemed to have found the magic key which could reactivate so many patients' self-healing ability. After a year or so, though, it became clear to her that the secret ingredient was enabling people to become fully and authentically true to themselves. She realized she was witnessing genuine spiritual healing. Gradually putting the pieces together, Rosy discovered that many people were living in circumstances that crushed the spirit, leaving them de-motivated or just lost. So many people are only half-alive, either leading a life dominated by the values, wishes and needs of others, or simply never being encouraged to live out their passion or purpose. She then grasped that the first step in healing any illness was to rekindle the 'inner fire', helping each person to discover what it is that really sparks them up and gives them a sense of purpose.

Over the 20 years Rosy has been exploring these concepts, scientific evidence has appeared to explain this phenomenon. This has come through discoveries in the area of PNI – Psychoneuroimmunology. This science was born with the discovery by Dr Candace Pert of the neuro-peptide, or informational substance, known as endorphin. From there, scientists went on to discover a further 200 tiny messenger chemicals for which there are receptors in both the brain and all tissues of the body. These discoveries changed the face of medicine and our understanding of human physiology for ever. No longer could the mind and body be seen as separate. Now, we could understand how these 'molecules of emotion', as Rosy calls them, mediate all the links between mind, body and spirit.

Going deeper into the study of PNI and what makes us ill, the findings are universal. Our immune system and healing and repair mechanisms crash when we experience loneliness, isolation or stress that we perceive beyond our control, and also when we repress or bottle up our feelings. Rosy began to understand how the holistic synthesis of spiritual revival, emotional release, the nurturing generated by gentle therapeutic techniques, and the deep inner calm produced through meditation and relaxation were having their effect.

Through the 1980s and 1990s, more thrilling scientific evidence came to light. Dr Steven Greer showed that women were 60 per cent more likely to survive breast cancer if they had a fighting spirit than if they felt helpless and hopeless. Professors Spiegel and Fawzy in the US showed that giving emotional support to people with cancer could double their survival time and revive their immune systems. Cardiologist Dr Dean Ornish showed that lack of love and intimacy were key factors in coronary artery disease, as were poor diet and lack of exercise. He found that support groups and stress reduction, when combined with a healthy diet and exercise, could actually reverse coronary artery disease.

Even more radical was the finding by Dr Lesley Walker that women who visualized their chemotherapy curing them had a 17.5 per cent survival advantage 13 years after the treatment than women who did not. Here was evidence of the immense power of the mind.

Today, there are thousands of studies showing that when we are in a happy, loving, enthusiastic state, our body functions optimally. There is of course always the exception to the rule, so we have to look into the chemical and genetic causes. We also know quite clearly that our immune system functions best when we are proactive, empowered and in control. So yes, it is vital to feed the body with healthy food, stop poisoning ourselves with cigarettes, alcohol and other toxic chemicals, take regular exercise and keep fit. But equally important is to take heed of your state of mind, and to address any congested emotional history, present pressures or fears.

All this depends first and foremost on coming into what Rosy calls 'a loving relationship' with our self, really learning to nurture ourselves at all the levels of body, mind, spirit and environment. Far too many of us have been brought up experiencing abuse, neglect and pressure. So many of us now hurtle through our lives, trying to meet myriad deadlines to achieve entirely artificial goals which are ultimately meaningless. Inevitably, if we care for ourselves this badly, our relationships with others will be unsatisfying too, and ultimately our relationship with life will become dull and lacklustre.

For Rosy Daniel, the real joy of working as an Integrated Medicine physician is helping individuals, bit by bit, to remove all the forces that are inhibiting or choking their life force, gradually re-kindling their creative fire until it is ablaze. She says: 'We must replace the negative and inhibiting voices of the past with positive, life-affirming, loving and encouraging voices empowering us to have a go, take a risk and be our full uninhibited selves. It really is that simple – and that hard.' See www.healthcreation.co.uk to read about Rosy's recommended ground-breaking natural medications.

Homeopathy – A Brief History

Samuel Hahnemann practiced medicine in the late 1700s, a time when large quantities of highly toxic substances, including mercury, arsenic and sulphur, were used to treat diseases that were rampant in those days, such as venereal disease.

Realizing that these treatments often killed rather than cured, Hahnemann began to experiment by diluting these poisons until he was no longer using material quantities yet was still curing his patients. He discovered that by noting what symptoms a healthy person exhibited when taking a substance, he could then match the remedy when the person was ill, returning them to a state of health. To put it simply, Hahnemann discovered that 'like cures like'. Thus homeopathy was born.

Homeopathic remedies do not have toxic side effects, because they consist of only a minute amount of active ingredients. Homeopaths examine the symptoms a patient is manifesting, but they also look at the things that frighten a person and whether the person is warm or cold temperature-wise. Homeopaths look at the whole story – the body and spirit. They examine the family history of disease, the psychological aspects, the patient's sleep patterns and diet. By collating all this information, the homeopath is able to identify the remedies that are most likely to help to alleviate or change the symptoms of imbalance that a patient is revealing.

Homeopathic remedies are made from all types of substances – from vegetation to snake venom – from the animal and mineral kingdoms and even from man-made substances. Practically anything that is used by humans can be turned into a remedy, even chemicals and other pollutants. They are, however, diluted to such an extent that there is nothing left of the original material – that is, they are sub-molecular. But the remedy absorbs the energy/vitality of that substance through the process of dilution in water. There is evidence that water retains the memory of substances that pass through it and is a very powerful conduit in its own right.

The oft-heard assertion by conventional medical practitioners that there is no scientific evidence for homeopathy completely ignores 250 years of clinical evidence of it working in practice.

Because pharmaceutical drugs can so often be toxic and have poisonous side effects – thalidomide being but one obvious example – they have had to be tested very carefully before being approved for use. Homeopathy does not use anything toxic, so it does not need to be tested in the same way, although the remedies are tested on volunteers in a carefully controlled system.

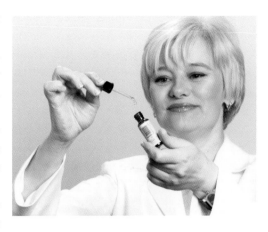

Lyndsey Booth, LCPH, MARH, worked for 17 years as a solicitor in the City and in local government. Having discovered homeopathy, after having children she gave up law and trained intensively for two years to qualify as a homeopath.

Homeopathy can aid people to change and transform their mental and emotional state in a fundamental way. It can help someone move from a place of despair to a dynamic frame of mind. However, there are many different ways of practicing homeopathy. Classical homeopaths, for example, emphasize the mental and emotional state and generally expect that physical symptoms will be the last thing to be changed. More eclectic practitioners use other tools such as diagnostic machines, herbs, dowsing and kinesiology to support their practice.

While recognizing the huge leaps people can make on a psychological level, it is also necessary to use homeopathy to support people going through this process on a physical level to underpin the changes.

How Complementary Practitioners Work

If you have chosen a therapy that is both diagnostic and prescriptive, such as homeopathy, naturopathy, iridology or ART, a very thorough case history will be taken. As a result, you may be given remedies or work to do along with recommended do's and don'ts.

If you are having a specific treatment, such as osteopathy, acupuncture or reflexology (or any form of body work), a case history is sometimes taken, however the emphasis is on the application and, thereafter, the feedback.

I could write an entire book on the myriad feedback I have had on the subject of complementary practitioners. Suffice to say that even though there are those who come across as know it alls with enormous egos or who are rude or give bad advice, the majority of people I have spoken to tell me they have derived immense help and advice from complementary medicine.

The best way to approach complementary medicine is to derive as much information as you can about the way the practitioner works and their experience. Then, once you are satisfied, learn as much as you can about yourself from them and don't waste time putting up barriers that demand they prove themselves to you. Equally, do not assign all power to that practitioner.

Concentrate on the resolutions you want and ask as many questions as you feel are necessary, so that you can be as independent in the management of your health, and as unreliant on the sort of medical treatment that can be invasive to your body, as possible. It is unlikely that any one practitioner will answer all your concerns – indeed be suspicious if someone makes rash promises. Even when you do get results, you have to be the judge as to when their effectiveness has run its course. Also make sure you understand what practitioners are recommending in terms of supplements and medication as sometimes they will work and sometimes they won't. If you fulfil your part of the relationship, remembering to factor in any existing emotional scenarios that may slow the process down, you will have mastered the 'how' of successfully getting results from this arena.

CASE STUDY – MAGDA'S STORY

Magda had never liked her stomach. It was a no-go zone as far as she was concerned. This affected not only how she looked but her breathing as well, which was very shallow.

As she was planning to have a baby, this was an area I focused on with Magda. However, whenever we did specific breathing exercises together, she found it very difficult and would become irritated and angry.

This reactionary approach to taking care of herself and doing the necessary work to bring about positive change was a pattern of Magda's. Up until her early forties, Magda all but ignored taking care of herself. She smoked, drank a glass or more of wine every night, and other than a few short spurts of cardiovascular exercise and upper body weight training, avoided the gym and exercise. The turning point for Magda came, as it does for many women, when she wanted to conceive.

Like many women her age, she had difficulty conceiving naturally. Initially Magda went to a homeopath to get pregnant but did not have any success; however, she later conceived using IVF. Towards the end of her pregnancy she became overdue and the doctors wanted her to be induced. Unhappy with this, Magda went to an acupuncturist who said he would not only bring on the birth but would tell her the sex of the baby beforehand.

Predictably, neither experience with complementary approaches resulted in the desired outcome. Magda approached homeopathy and acupuncture in the same reactionary way that she approached her body and health. I've seen this many times. It's almost like individuals expect some mystic or magical element in complementary medicine to immediately override years of continuing bad lifestyle choices. You can't just dive into anything without preparation and expect problems to be miraculously solved.

As with taking up exercise, timing is essential in incorporating complementary medicine so that you stand a good chance of benefiting from it. Not every practitioner is going to have the inclination or expertise to address your lack of care in areas like diet and exercise, or refer you to someone who may be more appropriate. Once I explained this to Magda, she was able to move on successfully and get value from complementary approaches.

If you have had a bad experience or simply haven't derived any results from one individual practitioner, communicating and giving feedback is imperative. It is also very important to check that you yourself have not contributed to a negative outcome. Whatever the experience, don't be put off from trying other practitioners.

CASE STUDY – CAROLE'S STORY

In my late twenties, I was introduced to an acupuncturist who charged a lot of money and was said to be brilliant. Apart from having an intense fear of needles, I was open to the experience. I went three times and derived no benefit whatsoever. It's true I didn't particularly warm to this practitioner as an individual, but I've never let that get in the way of deriving value.

When, 12 years later, a friend suggested I go to a local Chinese acupuncturist as I was emotional, spotty and generally not feeling well or looking great, I turned my nose up, saying I'd already tried acupuncture and it didn't work for me. But she persuaded me to go with her and after a 45-minute treatment – at a much lower cost than it had been all those years ago – I was pleased I'd gone. Two days later, my skin had completely cleared up and I felt great. Ever since then, whenever I feel the need, very sporadically, I go and see Michael at the Formosa Clinic and I always leave with positive results.

Conclusion

When you think about it, regaining your health is like renovating a house. There is a certain order in which things must be done, there are different experts whose help you must rely upon, and there are aspects that you as the owner must learn about and handle. You have to stay with the project until it ends and the house is just as you want it to be. Once the major renovations are finished, maintenance and refining are all that is left to oversee. It's the same with your health. If your body is overworked, stressed and/or near collapse, it's time to renovate. You can no longer just throw on a fresh coat of paint to try to maintain appearances.

A good place to start is to have a full medical, asking for any extra medical diagnostic tests that may be useful. Complementary therapists can help you with the planning, the wiring and the general overview, making sure everything within your structure is working together cohesively. Registering with a good, reputable homeopath, both for you and the rest of the family, is a sensible thing to do. And, if there are any mysteries or complications to do with your present health or well-being, cutting-edge therapies such as ART, Electronic Gem Therapy or specialized Chinese medicine amongst others can help uncover long-experienced physical and medical problems.

Food Matters

4

I LOVE FOOD. I CAN EAT ENDLESS amounts and I love both sweet and savoury food. I wish I could follow this by saying: 'and nothing affects my weight and well-being'.

I have come across very few people with worse eating habits than I had. The first 20 years of my life were filled with eating junk food. Other than potatoes, no vegetables found their way into my home, let alone my mouth. Fish was a rude word, and drinking water was for idiots.

I was (and still am) a chocoholic. When I do something bad, I do it really, really well. At my worst, I ate up to 50 chocolate biscuits a day and between six and 12 bars of chocolate at the same time, all washed down with three or four pints of full-fat milk, ice-cold from the fridge, with cheese and onion crisps interspersed to loop me back into wanting something sweet. And I haven't even told you yet what I ate at mealtimes…

What happened to me as a result? I got fat. I piled on three stone in my early twenties, which, for my frame, was a lot. I developed acne, chronic candida and fatigue syndrome, and was generally a mess. I did everything I could to deal with my problems except tackle my food intake. But my body wasn't having any of it, and just kept displaying all the signs of my self-destructive behaviour. So what's my point? It's that you can have the best complementary medicine, massage, colonic irrigation, communicational, attitudinal and NLP skills, you can take every supplement in the book and meditate all day, but if you don't get your food and liquid consumption right, you are wasting your time and your money.

Whether you like it or not, nutrition plays an enormously important role in your life. It affects the shape and feel of your body, your sexuality and self-confidence, your body odour and your skin. It can alter your emotional reaction, which in turn affects the way you think and behave. All this has a major influence on your ability to concentrate as well as the general running of every system in your body, including your cholesterol and blood pressure levels, hormones, metabolism, bowel function and digestive system.

What's The Crux Of The Problem?
What we have been left with is a tug of war between wanting to get rid of our weight and health problems, yet resenting or feeling lazy about having to do

what is necessary to attain that. For most of us, our weight, energy levels and general sense of well-being leave much to be desired.

In order to look, feel and be totally well and to have a clear mind, it is essential to understand the blocks and negative thoughts that prevent you from doing what is necessary to create and maintain that feeling of well-being and fitness. Our emotions are constantly changing: in women, PMS, as well as many other predicaments, can bring on depression and bingeing; for men, achieving their goals and proving themselves to their peers, whether consciously or otherwise, can pressurize them to keep up where food and drink are concerned. Self-esteem quickly dissolves when you put on weight and inches; your complexion becomes poor; your hair loses its gloss and your eyes lose their sparkle. No wonder people get depressed, bad tempered and anxious.

In the modern quest to find the perfect weight-loss regime, we have missed the point entirely. With obesity rates and illness at an all-time high, we either don't realize or don't care how much our eating habits are contributing to these problems. If our children aren't suffering from severe weight and obesity problems by the time they are six years old, they're likely to be suffering from a whole host of other illnesses such as asthma, eczema, constant mucus membrane problems affecting their ears, nose and throat, stomach disorders and multiple allergies. We're basically making each new generation's life a nightmare. If they are like this at such a young age, what on earth is it going to be like as they get older? The only way this legacy will change is for us to put into place a good system of nutrition that works for life, one that is in harmony with the seasons, and takes account of your energy levels, state of health, and every aspect of your physical and lifestyle needs and restrictions.

• The UK has the most overweight population in Europe – 46 per cent of men and 32 per cent of women are overweight.

What makes it so hard to eat properly is the huge choice of fast and rich foods, with sweet shops, patisseries and coffee shops on practically every street. Peer pressure at work and with friends, eating and drinking to be sociable, placating children through sugar and treats is literally killing us. Even when we go away, we feel we have to sample the local delights and drink our way through the holiday as some sort of reward for all our hard work. Alcohol and food are treated either as a reward, a comfort or an escape, depending on whether we feel happy or sad. It is easy to put the onus on government bodies, educational authorities and parent-teacher associations to make changes in schools; however, it will not be soon or thorough enough to give you what you need right now.

The quality of what we eat and where it is sourced from is of vital importance. The message that losing weight is the key factor in dealing with all weight issues and often other health-related problems is distracting our attention from what really matters and is diluting the importance of optimum nutrition for all.

A woman came up to me at work and asked me whether a particular diet would be good for her husband in order to lose weight quickly. I replied that unless he was going to stop eating foods that were fatty, mucus-forming, full of sugar and generally stressful to his heart, liver and kidneys, the diet wouldn't be any use to him. If, however, he did extract the rubbish from his life he wouldn't need to go on a fad diet.

Eating for the health of your organs and the capability of your digestive system, plus incorporating organic and biodynamic produce whenever possible, are key factors for good health. If your system is strong there is barely anything your body shouldn't be able to cope with in moderation. Allergies to foods decrease when you get the rubbish out of your body so that you can build up every system and organ to their natural state of strength and immunity.

When Did The Rot Set In?

Over the past 200 years, the content of the Western diet has dramatically changed. The Industrial Revolution led people away from the countryside into the cities, with an accompanying higher demand for food supplies. Newly developed manufacturing processes refined the food and began to increase the sugar and fat content to improve flavour and texture. Salt was also added as a preservative and flavouring. Foods began to be processed for preservation purposes, produced in large quantities and developed to suit changing taste preferences, but the new refined foods had deficiencies in vitamins, minerals and fibre.

Perhaps the single largest change in our diet over recent decades has been the inexorable rise of sugar, both as a main and as a hidden ingredient. From barely anything, consumption of sugar has risen to over 25 per cent in the modern diet, with the sugar industry pressing for that figure to be raised to 30 per cent or more. We also eat on average between 10 and 20 times more salt than our body requires on a daily basis.

Nutritional Deficiencies Worldwide

The change from relying on wild foods to domesticated and intensively farmed ones has had enormous implications for our health and the health of the animals and crops we are breeding and harvesting. Cultural diets all around the world are now showing patterns of nutritional deficiencies.

For example, in India, the development of and dependence on polished rice has led to the exclusion of other foods and therefore nutrients. A lack of foods rich in beta-carotene and vitamin A has meant that India has the highest rates of nutritional blindness in the world. Removing the nutrient-rich husk from the rice grain has led to an increase in the diseases beriberi and pellagra.

In Japan, the intake of fat has risen in the last 30 years from 10 per cent of the overall diet to 30 per cent. With this increase, there has been an almost identical surge in the rate of heart disease, as well as increases in height and changes in facial and body type.

Life Since The War

Before the Second World War, food was still mainly based around what could be grown and sourced locally and seasonally. That changed dramatically after the war,

• Following present trends, obesity will soon replace smoking as the greatest cause of premature loss of life in developed countries.

ending up with what we now have — access to global produce, enabling greater choice than ever before, but at what cost? During the war, the pharmaceutical industries worked hard to produce weapons and chemicals for the war effort. Afterwards, attention turned to food production, with the resulting explosion in pesticides, herbicides, antibiotics and fertilizers. And that's before we've mentioned what goes into the food after it has been harvested — preservatives, flavourings, colourings; all sorts of chemical newcomers for our bodies to deal with.

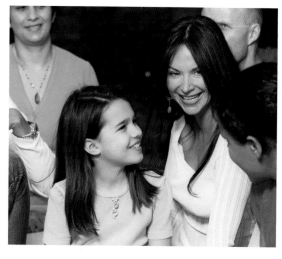

What goes hand-in-hand with this abundance of choice is that the nutritional content of what ends up on our plates has probably never been lower. And although we are told that each chemical is safe, there is clearly an impact that all the chemicals put together are having — not just in our bodies, but in the soil, on the fruits and vegetables, and the animals who are ingesting the same produce. It all adds up to one huge chemical time bomb.

Good nutrition can start at any age. Sarah Carolides' daughter Natasha enjoys what she eats without feeling deprived.

Before You Pick Up Another Diet Book

There are many misconceptions about what comprises healthy eating. The food manufacturers who have jumped on the 'healthy eating' bandwagon mislead us into thinking that buying tinned, packaged or ready-made meals with reduced or zero sugar or fat equals healthy eating. In general, there is very little real understanding of nutrition, either of what our bodies need or of the chemicals contained in both packaged and fresh foods — all of which have a major effect on our physical dysfunctions and weight problems. Seductive advertising is simply not to be believed.

When you and I think of a diet, there are several things that turn us away from a simple understanding and enjoyment of healthy eating. We tend to think only about what we cannot have, and that drives us towards resentment and depression. We inevitably give in to temptation and often end up eating double the quantity we would have done. Having fallen, we are upset with ourselves and angry too. It's simply too easy to think: 'To hell with it, it probably won't work anyway'. Then it's back to our old habits — or even worse. The end result is that even if you are really strict when on 'The Diet' and are successful in losing weight, once off the diet, nine out of 10 people find that within two months they've put the weight back on and are back to square one or worse.

Diets simply do not work. They are unrealistic, unhealthy, boring and traumatic, especially when you can't stick to them. Anyone who promises a quick-fix diet or forces you to change your diet so radically you won't be able to sustain it for longer than a few weeks is just wasting your time.

Dieting starves the body, slowing down the metabolism. Instead of burning up stored fat, the body gets used to working on fewer calories and readjusts itself to that level. If a dieter then increases his or her calorie intake even slightly, the extra calories will join other fat stores because the body's slowed-down metabolism will no longer require them. It's a vicious circle.

Contributing Factors To Weight Issues

Nine times out of 10, people wanting to lose weight have underlying general health issues. These may include a leaky gut, candida, irritated skin, bad breath, bowel disorders or exhaustion – the list is endless. To go on a diet or regime without taking that and your medical history into account will be detrimental to any unwanted conditions and also your desire to lose weight.

Nine Lives

You have nine lives when it comes to losing weight – in your twenties, you can binge and crash-diet to alarmingly fast results at both ends of the scale. When you get into your thirties, the backlash of any health issues or physically detrimental behaviour will have weakened your immune system without you necessarily realizing. So you still get results, but it's just that little bit harder. By the time you are 40, you've used up your nine lives and suddenly you hit a brick wall. By now your body is exhausted, your hormonal system is changing, and your body won't respond to the usual tactics. Nobody is too young to read this – teenagers and anyone in their twenties can stop the rot setting in before it's too late.

The Glycaemic Index

One of the biggest problems worldwide, which is also the most common contributory factor to the problem of excess weight, is a blood sugar imbalance due to our addiction and reliance on sugar in all its forms. This includes alcohol, cigarettes, cereals, sweets and all carbohydrates (even the good ones if they are ingested in too large a quantity). Until recently calorie counting was seen as essential for weight management; however, what scientists came to realize is that the sugar content of a food is far more relevant. As is the amount of acidic nutrient-starved food we often ingest.

The Glycaemic Index or GI measures how rapidly carbohydrates are absorbed into the bloodstream, causing the blood glucose level to rise, which then stimulates a rise in the level of insulin. Certain foods can be measured independently, and then assigned their own number on the Glycaemic Index. The scale runs from 0 to 100, with pure glucose scoring 100. High GI foods are rapidly absorbed and cause a large rise in blood sugar levels. Low GI foods release their glucose gradually and therefore have little effect on blood sugar levels. To allow a slow diffusion of energy through the body, four to five small meals a day are recommended rather than three large ones, thus helping to eliminate peaks and troughs of blood sugar, tiredness and alertness. Although some people find that eating more meals each day only increases their desire to eat more as they are thinking about food the whole time, others find it revolutionary.

Remember, the GI list is a guide to relative effects of different carbohydrate foods on blood glucose levels. As it is only a guide, individuals may react differently to individual foods and combinations.

Why Do Most Popular Diets Fail?

Each year we are inundated with the latest weight-loss programmes — almost all are based around losing dramatic amounts of weight in a few days or weeks. What they don't tell you is that you will almost certainly put this weight straight back on the minute you come off the diet.

Counting Calories

If only life was that simple! Unfortunately, balancing calorie intake against output just doesn't work. Why? Because of your body's metabolism. Metabolism is the name for every process in the body that involves energy. We are all born with a certain genetic rate of metabolism, which goes some way towards explaining why some people seem to be able to eat a whole bag of doughnuts and still stay thin, whereas others just have to look at one and put three inches on their hips. However, what we do with our body, and what we feed ourselves with, can either speed up our metabolism or slow it down by as much as 40–50 per cent. Some people have a faster rate of metabolism than others — they were made that way — but all of us can influence our own metabolic rates just by changing our eating and exercise habits.

The raw materials that we provide the body with — protein, fat and carbohydrates — are broken down to release energy. The lack of even a few vitamins and minerals essential for these processes can have a disastrous effect on the body, which begins to explain why so many of us feel tired when we do not get enough healthy nutrient-packed foods to keep our energy levels flowing.

Carole and renowned naturopath and dietician Elizabeth Gibaud checking out the new, healthy alternatives to tea and coffee.

The worst thing you can do for your metabolic rate is to crash diet or go on a low-calorie diet. Once you reduce the number of calories below a certain level, your brain receives the message that you are starving. So, to save energy, it slows down the rate of metabolism by as much as 45 per cent. Unfortunately, when the calories start flooding back in when you break the diet, your metabolism stays low, and because it has just come through a period of starvation, the body piles on as many fat stores as it can in case you are going to starve it again. This explains why

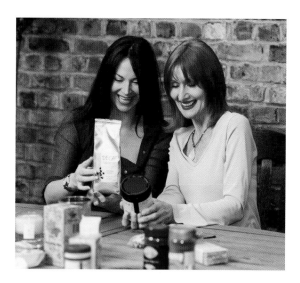

all the weight you lost during your two-week crash diet (and often more) piles straight back on the minute you come off it.

Another problem is that the human body is actually extremely intelligent. When you embark on any sort of badly planned calorie-restricted programme it is likely that you won't get enough of all the nutrients you need. Every day the body sends messages to the brain, telling you to eat more food to make up the lost nutrients – which is why so many people report huge cravings whenever they go on diets, and also why so many people binge the minute they stop the diet.

The Cardiovascular System

You may think that yo-yo or crash dieting bears no correlation to the cardiovascular system. However, have you stopped to think that the weight you are losing on these diets is a mix of fluid and glycogen released from lean muscle (because this is easier for the body to access rather than the actual fat that you are trying to lose)? And, of course, your heart is a muscle, and you don't want to lose lean tissue from any of your muscles, least of all your heart. Imagine then, if you are furiously working out as well, how much strain your heart will be under. As soon as you eat properly or go back to bad habits again, that water weight will go straight back on.

High-protein, Low-carbohydrate Diets

These types of diet have enjoyed enormous popularity in the last few years, mainly due to the impressive Dr Atkins' marketing machine. But beware. Too much protein in the system leads to the formation of toxic substances called ketones, especially if the body is being encouraged to burn protein to make fuel. The increased levels of ketones can induce a toxic bodily state called ketosis, which can be harmful, and is certainly unnatural. A further side effect of eating too much protein is that amino acids (which is what protein is made up of) are released into the blood. In order to neutralize these acids, the body needs to find some alkaline minerals – and it does this by leaching calcium, an alkaline molecule, out of the bones. Thus consuming too much acidic food of any kind, but especially dense animal proteins, can increase your risk of osteoporosis. This is only one example of a number of adverse reactions the body can suffer from.

Low-fat Diets

These diets are very popular, but the problem is that most people don't know the difference between good and bad fats. They simply cut out all fats and oils, and then wonder why they are feeling cold, depressed or their skin is dry. There are a number of fats that are absolutely essential to the body as they are needed to make hormones ... and it is hormones that keep us warm and aid our metabolism, while the fats plump up our skin. It is preferable to keep saturated fats (that's the animal kind) out of your diet, but you must make sure you keep up your intake of essential fats, which are found in seeds, wholegrains and fish.

Uniquely You

Be careful about what you are being told to do. It's a little like when you read your star sign – if you go through everyone's, you can probably relate to any of them. It is the same with diets. However, you have to take into account your own medical history: how your bowels are functioning, your everyday state of health, spots, energy levels and output, eczema, thyroid function, stomach problems, flatulence and so on. It is vital that you remember that you are unique. What works for one person doesn't necessarily translate for another. For example, we know that pasta is a low GI food, yet the feedback nutritionists get all the time from clients is how they feel bloated and yet not necessarily satisfied when they've finished eating pasta. Or that they so love pasta that it becomes 70 per cent of their food intake and they are piling on the pounds. Take a baked potato, which is supposed to be a high GI food and is also part of the nightshade family, and yet when people have used an organic baked potato as one of their main meals in a day with a light salad, they are completely satisfied and there is no bloating. After a couple of weeks of including this in their diet, plus the right amount of protein and green vegetables in another meal, people found they had lost weight, their cravings had gone and they still had loads of energy. Everyone is different, so the more self-knowledge you have the more successful you will be. How you feel when you eat and the conditions with which you are eating that food, for example sitting down and not on the hop, will alter the function, process and assimilation that does or does not take place in your body.

Factors That Affect Weight And Health Issues

There are a number of factors that can affect weight. These include:

• Hypothyroidism (underactive thyroid): lowers metabolism so energy is stored not burnt.

Action: test thyroid function with the basal temperature test; exercise increases metabolic rate; reduce the following foods in your diet: soya, beans, brassicas; avoid fluoride; include intake of iodine-rich foods such as seaweed and/or kelp supplement.

• Toxicity/poor liver function (as in food intolerances): toxins are stored in fat cells away from more sensitive tissue, these fat cells therefore become very hard to shift.

Action: follow a short cleanse; address nutrient deficiencies; drink more water; minimize intake of toxins (alcohol, caffeine, pollution); gentle exercise; to improve liver function use herbal remedy milk thistle; take a green food to increase the alkalinity of your system; check with a naturopath or homeopath which tissue salts would be good for you; use steam or sauna treatments after exercise as the process of sweating is one of the best ways of eliminating chemical toxins from fat cells.

Other contributing factors to look at include irregular bowels, lack of sleep, medication, travelling, injuries, trauma, stress and hormone imbalances.

Parasites

A parasite is an organism that exploits another living organism in order to feed and grow. In most cases, the parasitic process causes harm to the person, whether through the actual removal of nutrients (which may include partially digested material, blood and so on), by causing disease or by carrying other diseases and bacteria into the body.

Parasites can be broadly sorted into two categories: ecto- and endoparasites. Ectoparasites (ecto = outside) do not live within the body, but visit and feed on people (or other living organisms). The main danger is that in the process of feeding on the person's blood, they may introduce other bugs to the body. Examples of ectoparasites include mosquitoes (malaria), tsetse flies (sleeping sickness) and culex (West Nile virus).

Endoparasites live and feed within the person, the majority either in the gut or blood system. There are some parasites that live at least part of their life cycle within body tissues such as the lymph nodes, muscle, brain and eye. Organisms that live in the blood, such as the malarial parasite, have distinct and obvious symptoms, and a GP will quickly be able to test for them.

A plethora of parasites inhabit the human gut, ranging from microscopic single cell organisms to worms several feet long. Parasites are often thought of as a tropical problem, but this is a misconception. It's estimated that a considerable percentage of the population are infected as a result of contaminated water, food or direct contact. Many people will carry parasitic infections at a sub-clinical level for years, with the parasite feeding, reproducing and affecting their health. Bloating, flatulence, an inability to absorb nutrients or a weak immune system are major reasons for intolerances, allergies, and weight that you cannot lose regardless of exercise and diet.

Fungi

Fungi and yeasts are multi-celled plant parasites that thrive in warm, damp, moist environments. Rather like a primitive vegetable, fungi can be found in the air, soil and water and on plants. There are millions of different types, the most familiar being mushrooms, yeast moulds and mildews.

Common fungal infections include: candida, vaginal candidiasis, oral thrush, athlete's foot, ringworm (not a worm but a fungus), fungal nail infections and tinea barbae (known as Barber's itch).

Candida is very common nowadays, and species of candida are normally found in the mouth, throat, digestive tract and vagina. Unfortunately, this fungus can produce disease in any part of the body, and in very bad cases can cause systemic infections of the brain and heart.

To fight a candida infection, it helps to cut out certain foods that can feed it. A candida infection can also be the cause of intolerances to certain foods and these should be limited or eliminated to give the intestinal walls a chance to heal and rebalance the flora and fauna in these areas. These foods usually include: yeast products, bread, cakes, pastries, some pasta, mushrooms, potatoes, fruit, chocolate, corn, wine and sugar. Before removing these items from your diet, check with a practitioner. Everyone is different and each person should be tested and advised nutritionally. The Novo test and ART practitioners are able to test for the food intolerances that contribute to candida.

Fungi have been with us for thousands of years and have cohabited with the human species since we began. We eat fungi and enjoy them, they live within us and are necessary, but they can get out of balance and cause problems

The Bowels

When the bowels are not emptied daily, the faeces in the bowel creates toxic fluid and gas that can invade the intestinal tract, digestive system, central nervous system, glandular structure, skin and breath. You may experience heartburn, flatulence, possibly bleeding gums, mouth ulcers and cold sores. Your skin may be cloudy, spotty, dull and puffy; your hair may look greasy and lifeless. The eyes are often dull and red and your head may be thick and heavy, sometimes with appalling headaches and migraine. Brain chemistry can alter and leave you feeling anxious, depressed, frustrated, angry or moody. Sex becomes a turn-off – you feel uncomfortable with a full bowel, wind and gas. Irregular bowel movements can also be a major contributing factor in weight problems.

There is simply no alternative but to have a clean, clear bowel. Not convinced? Equate the faeces in your bowel with some meat left on a dish in the kitchen for 48 hours. How would it look and smell after this time?

The 'perfect' stool should leave the body comfortably and fully, be fairly bulky and very light in weight; it should float in the water. If this is not the case adjust your fibre intake accordingly; eat more if the stool is hard, less if the stool is loose. Also make sure you make time to go to the toilet so you do not rush it.

The Stomach – Acid And Ulcers

Most people do not realize that their stomach contains very powerful hydrochloric acid (HCl). This acid is so strong it would burn the skin or clothing. But in the stomach – which is protected by a thick mucus coating – HCl aids both digestion and sterilization. Firstly, it acts by killing off any potentially hazardous microbes and bacteria in our food, protecting us against food poisoning and infections. Secondly, it acts to break down the food, especially proteins, so that they can be absorbed further down the digestive tract.

It is often said you are what you eat, but it would be truer to say that you are what you absorb. You can eat the best diet in the world, but unless you are able to digest it and fully absorb the nutrients, you won't be getting the benefits. Also, in order to digest food, the body needs oxygen, which is why it's important to sit down and relax while eating. If you eat while working, moving around or focusing your energy on other matters, oxygen will be diverted to needs other than digestion and the process will slow down.

As they get older, many people find they have problems with digestion, primarily heartburn and indigestion, bloating, belching and flatulence. This can often be due to the fact that with age, levels of HCl tend to decline.

Aside from age, there are other factors that affect our ability to digest and absorb food:

• Stress. Long- or short-term stress can affect the amount of stomach secretions and also the length of time food is in the stomach. Most of us know the sensation of a knotted stomach; it is feelings like this and anxiety that can affect the digestive process in a negative way.

• Overeating and/or eating too quickly. This slows down digestion or causes food to pass through the system without being digested fully, thus impairing nutrient absorption.

• Irregular eating. This disturbs the natural rhythms of the digestive system.

• Eating late at night, or eating when you are suffering exhaustion and any emotional stress, anger or worry.

• Sensitivities. Many people are sensitive to certain foods even though the symptoms may not be obvious. If a reaction is happening internally, digestion will be impaired in various ways, either causing a chemical reaction which can result in indigestion, headaches, fatigue and lack of concentration, or in an external way, showing as a rash or sensation such as nausea or itching.

Antacids

People who believe they produce too much acid tend to relieve their discomfort after meals by taking antacids – alkaline products designed to neutralize the amount of acid in the stomach. In fact, the problem usually lies in the stomach lining. Years of eating irritants and poor food, along with a stressful life, can cause tiny lesions in the lining, allowing a bacteria called Helicobacter pylori to take hold and make the lesions worse. Once this happens, even normal levels of stomach acid can irritate the lining and cause discomfort and pain. All antacids do is relieve the symptoms by neutralizing the acid. But this in itself causes more problems, firstly because the stomach is now not able to break down foods and kill bacteria, and secondly because the stomach needs to keep the acid at a certain, very precise, level. Once the brain receives a message that the acidity of the stomach has gone down, it will work harder to produce more acid next time, causing more discomfort.

Some common medications such as aspirin or anti-inflammatory drugs can also irritate your stomach.

Implementing Healthy Nutrition

One of the reasons we find it so hard to stick to any healthy eating plan is that we don't set up our environment at home or at work with the right foods, liquids and, where appropriate, supplements. Getting rid of the temptations that are so easy to reach for, especially when your resolve is even slightly dented, is crucial.

Shopping for food is another key factor. To get into the habit of buying your food correctly, ordering the food to suit your needs and tastes at a restaurant, and communicating to friends and colleagues when being entertained, are key elements. There's no use starting to eat healthily if you're going to stop-start because of social commitments and not wanting to lose face.

How To Shop In Supermarkets

It is easy to shop healthily at all the major supermarkets nowadays. Almost all of them have good organic sections, and if your local one doesn't, make sure you ask why not! Head for the fresh fruit and vegetables, but try and keep in mind what is 'fresh' and in season. Ideally, you want to buy food that is as fresh and packed full of nutrients as possible. Avoid so-called 'fresh foods' that have travelled halfway around the world and taken three weeks to arrive. Don't buy ready-made meals, which are full of sugar and sodium. Frozen foods are better than cook-chill alternatives that have probably sat in the cabinet for three days leaching vitamins. And if you are really pushed for time, do all your ordering on the internet and have it delivered to your door.

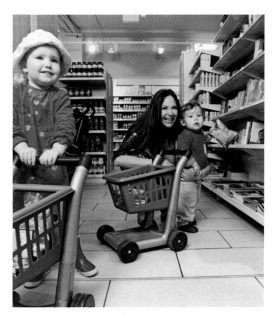

Carole at Planet Organic, with kids running around helping their parents with the shopping.

Avoid shopping on autopilot, sailing along the aisles and choosing the same products every week. Never go shopping on an empty stomach or when you feel cravings coming on. Also try to shop in places other than supermarkets, such as health food shops, greengrocers, fishmongers and farmers' markets. This will help you to avoid temptation and also increase your knowledge of different healthy food options. Choosing organic food helps to reduce the toxic burden of the environment on your body. Not only does the cocktail of hormones, pesticides and growth promoters in non-organic produce have to be detoxified by your liver, but they can accumulate in body tissues.

Check food labels and become more familiar with the terminology. Many everyday items such as bread have a long list of ingredients that would never be included in a homemade version. Compare the list on a packet of butter to that on a tub of margarine and you will see that butter is a much more natural product. Food manufacturers know that we are becoming more aware of our nutrition and they are becoming increasingly clever. Look out for the hidden sugar and substitute sweeteners. Sugar can be listed as dextrose, glucose, sucrose and fructose to name but a few. When checking labels look for those names ending in 'ose', which sadly in many products you will see more than once and often very high up on the list. Even in organic supermarkets the salt level is often high, both in ready-made foods and packaged food stuffs.

Sulphur dioxide is another ingredient found in drinks, foods and skin products and is a known irritant that can cause headaches and skin complaints, plus your healthy stomach bacteria does not respond well to it. Check every ingredient on the label and if there is something you are not sure of, leave it alone or look it up in Felicity Lawrence's book *Not On The Label* to identify whether the food should be in your basket or not. If you are avoiding wheat or dairy, read the labels very carefully. You will see that they both crop up everywhere, and often where you least suspect, especially in sauces and other packaged foods.

Where possible avoid tinned and processed foods. Foods that have been sitting in a tin can are not going to be the most nutritious, and if you check the use-by dates, you will see that they may have been in the can for years. Sometimes your lifestyle dictates that you need to buy these items on occasion, but again choose the organic options without added salt and sugar and that don't have quite as long a shelf life.

Whether or not you are following a weight-loss plan, avoid the low-fat, low-calorie options. Reducing the levels of fat or sugar means that these ingredients must be replaced with something else, and very often something of a chemical nature. Choosing whole foods invariably means they are naturally low in fat and sugar and the fats they contain are far more likely to be of the beneficial kind.

See www.lifesmart.co.uk for healthy food and drink shopping lists.

Eating Out

We eat out more than ever, for business, pleasure, a special occasion or because it saves having to cook. Temptations are usually rife and often impossible to resist, but there are many ways to make these outings healthier.

To begin with there is now a huge choice of restaurants serving the sort of food you can – and should – eat without feeling deprived: fresh grilled fish, lean meats, light soups and grain dishes, an immense variety of vegetables, salads and other good and delicious food. Drink mineral water with ice and lemon in a wine glass. Make the most of the opportunity to have all the good things you enjoy, without the effort of having to shop for them, cook and wash up.

However, be aware that a lot of restaurant dishes are overloaded with salt, oil and flour as well as sugar, sugar substitutes and more. Make a list of what you don't want to eat so that you can let the waiter or manager know when ordering, or call ahead and order giving any required information. They are used to requests, so don't use any excuses not to take advantage of doing this. If you don't want to drink alcohol, but are embarrassed, simply say you've had a stomach upset or better still get used to not bothering about what people think. Very soon they will drop the pressure and you will enjoy the freedom to drink only when it works for you or when you are really in the mood and not just as a matter of peer pressure or habit.

• Spending on organic foods exceeded £1.1 billion in 2003.

Remember, whatever you choose to eat, even if it's breaking your healthy regime, enjoy it and don't attach feelings of guilt to food, just make sure you continue with your healthy eating plan afterwards.

1. When going out for a meal eat a healthy snack before – not so much that your appetite is ruined, but just so you're not ravenous. An apple or some seeds and crudités is just enough to take the edge off your appetite and help you keep away from the bread basket and over eating.
2. Politely refuse the bread basket before they have a chance to put it down. If you do succumb, choose brown bread with (unsalted) butter not margarine.
3. As you should do at every meal, chew food thoroughly. This helps satisfy your taste buds and appetite and is essential for proper digestion. It also allows the brain time to register that you are eating and to savour and enjoy the flavours.
4. Fill up on vegetables. Any good restaurant should be able to prepare you a side order of steamed vegetables with a squeeze of lemon, some ground black pepper, garlic and whatever herbs you fancy. If you are on a weight-loss programme, choose green vegetables over carrots – potatoes do not count towards your vegetable quota as they are a main part of the meal.
5. Avoid creamy sauces, MSG (monosodium glutamate), highly salted or fried food. You are there to enjoy yourself, not to make yourself ill the next day.
6. If you choose to have dessert, make sure you really want it and enjoy it. If, however, you have told yourself you will skip dessert then don't have it and don't even bother looking at the dessert menu. Saying no automatically means that there won't be an opportunity for something to catch your eye only to weaken your resolve.
7. Sip liquid with your meal rather than 'washing it down' with huge gulps. Consuming too much liquid with food can dilute the digestive juices and impair digestion, leaving you bloated and lethargic.
8. Being entertained at other people's homes and reciprocating is another popular way of eating out. Often these are the hardest situations to be in. Not wanting to be rude or, alternatively, wishing to outdo previous hosts are the two major reasons why we fall down when trying to stick to a healthy regime. My advice is to always communicate ahead of time when you're the guest, and to serve up delicious healthy meals when it's your turn to cook, using it to set a new trend amongst your peers.

Acid And Alkaline Foods

Foods are classified as acid or alkaline, not because of their taste but according to the residue left after they have been metabolized in the body. Many people have a diet which is often composed of at least 80 per cent acid-forming foods, which creates an adverse overload on our blood and tissues.

Carole with the creator and owner of Planet Organic, Renee Elliott and her daughter, Jessica. Renee has had a profound effect and influence on raising both consumers' and retailers' awareness of the importance of organic food and healthy choices in complementary medicine and alternative skin products – from babies through to adults.

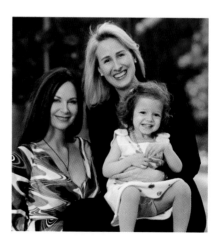

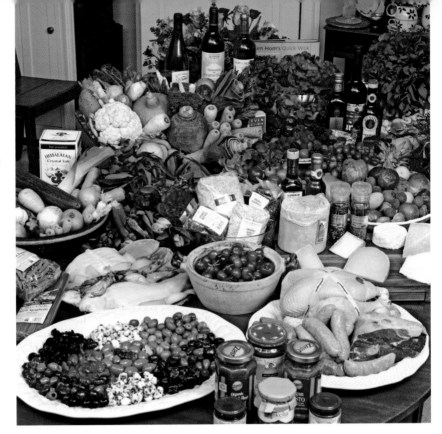

Contrary to what many people still believe, healthy eating doesn't have to be boring. You just have to broaden your knowledge of all the food products that are available to you.

The body tries to eliminate acid via the kidneys and bowel, with the overload taken out through the sinuses, other mucus membranes and skin. Ideally, for our systems to remain free of congestion, mucus and too much acidity, between 70 and 80 per cent of our food intake should be alkaline. In addition, having the correct balance of vitamins and minerals as well as the right essential fatty acids and amino acids to perform the required fat and protein functions will keep your system functioning optimally.

If you are suffering from a lack of sleep, overwork, worry, anger, jealousy, resentment, fear or apathy, this can turn food (including alkaline foods) acidic.

Go to www.lifesmart.co.uk for a full list of acid and alkaline foods.

Food Combining

Food combining is a way to attain easy, efficient digestion and to eliminate gastric upset. Due to our exhausting lifestyles and – for many – our depleted digestive systems, we often cannot cope with more than one concentrated food at a time. The main principle of this system of preparing meals is to eat simply and without combining too many substances at any one time. This may appear bothersome, time-consuming and of little value, but food combining is not new. It has been practised by many cultures for centuries, to good and often transformative effect.

If you choose to follow a food combining diet try to eat one starch-based meal and one protein-based meal a day, at least four hours apart. Avoid eating fruit in the morning and ideally do not eat other foods within a couple of hours of eating fruit. Your body requires energy first thing and the body cannot readily convert fruit while the digestive system is still sluggish from sleep. Fruit will not soak up the acids in the stomach either, unlike grains, nor will it give you adequate fuel at the start of the day. The exception to this rule is if it is summer or you are on holiday and the fruit is seasonal to the country you are in.

Following the guidelines on eating fruit within the food-combining chart (see www.lifesmart.co.uk) is extremely important as the body will respond better to breaking down the acids and absorbing the nutrients. As a general guideline the most important time to food combine is during your working week.

Organic And Biodynamic Produce

Many people view organic food as a luxury, thinking that it is a relatively new idea. In fact, up until the twentieth century organic whole foods were the foundation of everyone's diet. 'Progress' has brought with it convenience and fast food, and demand has been so great that our food is grown in chemically rich soil, treated with pesticides and insecticides and sprayed, preserved and injected with chemicals. Unless you buy organic or biodynamic meat, the animals will have been pumped full of antibiotics and growth hormones. So buying organic or biodynamic is the best thing we can do to minimize unwanted rubbish going into our bodies, and to give our system the fuel it needs to operate healthily.

• Over the past five years the sales of organic food have almost trebled.

Austrian philosopher Rudolf Steiner pioneered biodynamic farming in 1924 by encouraging farmers and soil scientists to choose not to follow the world into the widely promoted 'chemical future'. Even in 1924, there was a noticeable degradation in the quality of soil, seed, plant and animal life. Biodynamic farming is a worldwide, non-chemical agriculture movement which pre-dates 'organic' farming by two decades. However, biodynamic farming is about more than avoiding chemicals. It emphasizes ecological harmony and environmental sustainability with food that is grown with particular composts, preparations and natural activating substances to provide real nutrients to the land in order to yield high-quality, nourishing food.

If you use chemically grown fruit and vegetables, make sure you wash and scrub them well or peel them to avoid ingesting pesticides and other chemicals.

The Amount You Eat

The quantity of food you eat is very important. Your system must be balanced – if it is over- or under-filled your body is likely to react adversely. People who do not think constantly about their next meal (or eat more than they need) are often the healthiest because they respond to purely natural incentives to eat. This is not always easy to do because many of us have been brought up to leave a clean plate. Coupled with the fact that most of us enjoy eating and eat too quickly, resulting in large amounts being consumed at once, it is all too common for people to forget how much our bodies really require. Even when eating healthy foodstuffs we can easily overeat. Slowing down, chewing thoroughly and, most of all, listening to your body, not your head, are key to food working for you, not against you.

Whatever complaints you have, either weight- or healthwise, the times to eat that have the worst effect on your body are when you are upset, angry, tired, bored, jealous, rushing around or over-excited. This is because your nervous system starts working overtime, your breathing becomes irregular, and the muscles around the stomach and diaphragm go into spasm – all of which stop your digestive system from working properly. This can prevent the kidneys and gall bladder from getting rid of poisons efficiently and, depending on how badly you are affected by your emotions (no matter how alkaline and clean your food is), your body will turn what you have ingested into acid.

So be warned. Eating while in these states can make an existing complaint far worse than if you were in a normal, relaxed state of mind. Make sure that before you eat you are sitting down comfortably, breathing properly and are calm. Then eat only a small amount of something that is easy to digest.

Breakfast

Breakfast is extremely important, but you do not necessarily have to eat it the minute you get up. We usually overload our bodies with too much food at one sitting, especially late at night. Eating before you have flushed out the acids that have risen during the night can initially feel like a relief, especially if you have a headache or are feeling sluggish. However, eating straight after you wake up only pushes the acids back down into the digestive tract, increasing the toxins internally; it's only a matter of time before the headache and sluggishness reappear. What then follows mid-morning is the uncontrollable need for something salty or sugary (or both) to banish this feeling … and the rest of your day usually follows in the same vein.

A good way to start the day is to have one or two large mugs of hot water made from bottled water or Aquathin water system (see page 219). When drinking your hot water, you are likely to feel a pleasant sensation in the solar plexus and the rest of your digestive system, especially when the water begins to clear the toxins and waste, encouraging much-needed elimination.

Don't rush straight into eating unless you are honestly hungry; your body will let you know when you are really ready to have breakfast. Equally, if you skip breakfast or leave it too long, your metabolism will be disturbed and cravings will take over. Often people feel so good after drinking the hot water that going off to work and having their breakfast between 8 and 10am works well for them.

Go to www.lifesmart.co.uk for delicious breakfast ideas and recipes.

Eating Late

Don't do it! Your digestive system simply doesn't work efficiently after 8pm. If you cannot eat before then, choose something light on which to dine. People often feel tired in the morning as the body doesn't stop digesting just because you have decided to go to sleep. Waking up lethargic, full of mucus with foul-tasting breath, is the norm for many. Often this alone can be responsible for a person having problems with their weight and general well-being. Many people find that having a light supper early in the evening is excellent when trying to lose weight, as well as greatly benefiting energy levels as sleep will not be interrupted by having to digest food.

Three Square Meals A Day

The benefit of eating three regular meals a day is that your body is provided with a steady flow of energy. You should not experience a sinking of energy when called upon to perform tasks or make important decisions, but should be creative and satisfied with your output. Miss a meal and you may miss an opportunity or an important point in a meeting. Skipping lunch and compensating by eating a huge dinner is particularly self-defeating as your system simply cannot cope. Remember it takes approximately four to eight hours to digest a meal.

Five Meals A Day

Eating five smaller meals is especially beneficial for men and women dealing with blood sugar and digestive problems, cravings and major energy swings. Menopausal and pregnant women may also find that lighter, more frequent meals are a help. What you have to watch is that all your energy is not taken up with digestion. You will know if this is the case if you want to sleep all the time. Again, the success of eating in this way is down to you experimenting and making sure that your portions are not too large.

Vegetarian Diets

One of the most often-asked questions is: 'How do I get my protein if I am a vegetarian?' To get protein, always mix a grain with a legume (pulses), as whatever is nutritionally lacking in the grain will be made up in the legume. Sprinkling seeds and nuts out of the shell or a few almonds on most dishes will also ensure a healthy supply of protein. Beware of overeating dairy products to compensate for losing meat. Many vegetarian recipes use cheese, but use goat's or sheep's cheese and soya products where possible.

Another question is: 'Where do I get my calcium from if I'm not eating any dairy produce?' The best source of calcium is sesame seeds (in such things as tahini), plus dark green, leafy vegetables. Almonds are another good source and unlike some other nuts are easily digestible – grind them and add water to make almond 'milk'. Experiment with soya mince (which you can use to make sausages, pies and other traditional meat-based dishes if you really are missing meat) and tofu (use in curries and stews).

Bran and wholegrain wheat can block the absorption of minerals, particularly calcium, magnesium, iron and zinc, so take care not to overeat these foods. Remember that tea and coffee inhibit the absorption of iron and that iron deficiency can be a problem for vegetarians. Don't drink tea or any caffeine-based drink with meals – instead stick to water or herbal teas (fennel and peppermint aid digestion, and nettle is a rich source of iron).

If you are a vegan or vegetarian, a B12 vitamin supplement such as BioCare's sublingual B12 with vitamin C (see page 214), evening primrose oil, star flower oil or borage oil is invaluable. Vegetarian diets are low in vitamin B12 (although complete deficiency is rare) and it can be found in small quantities in dairy products, brewer's yeast and eggs.

Fasting, Cleansing And Healing

So many of us use food, alcohol and both pharmaceutical and recreational drugs to excess. This causes congestion and stagnation in the organs, tissues, circulation, lymph and cells. Detoxification is the process that can be used to eliminate all this and neutralize your internal system. It is used extensively by professionals to aid their clients in dealing successfully with serious and moderate illnesses and conditions. Ideally cleanses should be done seasonally so that the body becomes used to the process, regularly deleting any backlog that can cause unwanted conditions. Remember that your body also has a daily elimination cycle, if you allow it to, which takes place mainly at night and in the early morning, up until the time when you have breakfast.

When you feel yourself coming down with a cold or sore throat you can detox both internally and externally by taking Bioforce's C and F complex, gargling with pure sea salt or Himalayan salts (see page 205), ingesting a nutritious soup, bathing and then sleeping until you wake up the following morning fully restored. Likewise, if your bowel feels congested and your head and stomach are affected, give your digestive system a break by drinking only liquids, for example soup, and use gentle herbs to stimulate your colon, which will usually put you back on track. This is about you taking control, honing your ability to define, refine and act appropriately where any 'dis-ease' or malady is concerned.

It is important to detox only when your body is ready, so prepare yourself beforehand. Going from eating unhealthily and drinking alcohol, tea and coffee straight into fasting (and then reverting quickly back into your old habits) puts extra strain on your system. Secondly, fasting or eating just fruit and water for two or three days won't achieve a cleansed state. You can't correct and heal the body in so short a time. Only once you have been eating properly for at least two weeks and you feel strong and healthy as a result, can you do a vegetable and home-made soup cleanse. Don't fast when you are under stress, and make sure you get extra sleep and pampering so that your energy for work is not greatly impaired.

To really cleanse the body and combat weight and health problems, nutritionists will advise you to start by reducing, and then cutting out completely the following: wheat, yeast, salt, dairy produce (except, depending on your mucus production, possibly a twice-weekly dish of goat's or sheep's milk yoghurt with live cultures of acidophilus) tea, coffee, alcohol and all additives and preservatives. Most nutritionists will also suggest that you reduce your fruit intake, either asking you to cut it out for a period of time or to eat only soft fruits such as pears, nectarines and peaches, and limit them to two a day eaten on their own. Oranges, pineapple, grapefruit, tangerines, apples, grapes and bananas are usually omitted as these are known to create cravings or to ferment in the body. It's up to you whether you cut down your intake of these foods over a two-week period before eliminating them completely or not.

Whenever you decide to go on an elimination or detoxification programme, I strongly suggest you start it on a Friday evening so you have the weekend to get over the worst side effects. (If you are using this information to help you recover from a binge it could be any day of the week.)

Make your home as clean, comfortable and tidy as possible, with clean sheets on the bed and the chores done. Also make sure you have an adequate supply of water, BioCare's powdered acidophilus and bifidis to replace healthy gut bacteria, and their cranberry and acidophilus capsules for any sensations of cystitis (see page 214). Also have Biona's organic pure cranberry juice. It's probably best during a detox to have a period of time off your usual supplements so that your body has a complete break from routine. Rather than take pharmaceutical drugs, homeopathic remedies such as Nux vomica, Belladonna and Byronia are very effective remedies if your head and stomach are problematic in the first 48 hours, which is a normal occurrence during cleanses. Herbs, such as nettle and fennel, are great made up as herbal teas (tisanes) and add extra strength when flushing out your body's attackers. There are many other homeopathic and natural remedies which can be taken at this time to help fortify the liver and balance the thyroid (which controls your metabolism). The Organic Pharmacy (see page 209) provides a good guide to what you can have during these times. Enviva (see page 108) also have an unbeatable support programme of eliminators and liquid nutrient products and recommendations.

Drink lots of water at either hot or room temperature, including the tisanes. Bathing, steaming and sleeping, lymphatic drainage and particularly acupuncture will speed your system back to order and complete the cleansing process. Do not have any food apart from what has been suggested for your recommended regime.

If you have any medical conditions, are pregnant or taking medication, you must check first with your GP before you detox.

Make sure that when you finish your fast, you reintroduce yourself to eating with very light, easily digested foods such as soups, ungassy green vegetables, fish and baked potatoes. Until digestive health is restored no weight-loss plan, fast or cleanse will work in the long run without upsetting your metabolism, especially the older you get. What you actually need to learn to do is to encourage movement, freedom and elimination within the body – mobilizing the lymph, increasing blood circulation and opening up all the routes of elimination. In other words, the body needs to cleanse before it can absorb.

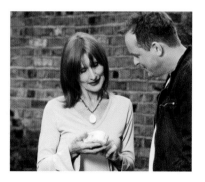

Elizabeth Gibaud advising Mike, who has already gone from 17 down to 13 stone, how he can improve his nutrition further.

Food Sensitivities And Allergies

Food sensitivity is extremely common. Without necessarily realizing it, people can become sensitive at any time to any substance. Sometimes you may get a rash or feel a little lethargic after eating certain foods. Discovering your food sensitivities can be a short-cut to solving your weight and health problems. Remember, people with food allergies don't have the immunity to deal with processed or junk foods, or with too many ingredients or seasonings, artificial colours or preservatives. If you have been correctly diagnosed and are eating the right quantity and quality foods, coupled with cutting reactive substances from your diet, a number of your sensitivities should cease, taking with them the headaches, apathy, lethargy and cravings. Variety is the key to a healthy diet – don't get stuck eating the same food every day, and don't starve yourself as that will only make your condition worse. Rotate your foods as much as possible, as sticking to one food regularly is one of the main reasons why people develop food intolerances or allergies. I had multiple sensitivities when I started out, and 90 per cent of them are no longer an issue. I now know exactly when I need to cut out certain foods, and that kind of self-knowledge is priceless. Getting through that 'tough stage' is the only way you will continue to achieve and maintain your results. Remember what you may be up against:

1. A lifetime of bad eating habits.
2. No nutritional education.
3. Your daily ups and downs and emotional problems – you can no longer use food to deal with these.
4. Addictions to tastes.
5. Cravings due to nutrient deficiencies.
6. Eating on the run.

There are many conflicting views surrounding food allergies and food sensitivities, the way they are diagnosed and their relevance to weight and health problems. But there are several factors, such as age, gender, genetics, stress, attitudes, pollens and environmental pollution that affect the presence of food sensitivities, intolerances and allergies.

Allergy Tests

Allergy tests can be very useful, but have been shown in some instances to be inaccurate. The Novo test works in a different way to other allergy and sensitivity tests as it looks for an inflammatory response to foods via the body's immune system. Utilizing state-of-the-art laser technology, this blood test can detect over 20,000 reactions to each and every food. Unlike other tests Novo does not look specifically at just one protein produced by the immune system called IgG, but at the body's complete white blood cell response. Looking for only IgG can lead to many false negatives, as this protein is only produced by the body in

• 45 per cent of people suffer from some kind of food intolerance.

response to a food when it has been fighting that food for three to four consecutive days. Therefore, if a person hasn't eaten a foodstuff regularly or before that four-day period, other intolerances will not be detected. By focusing on the body's whole white blood cell response rather than just a single protein the Novo test is able to pick up even the slightest of sensitivities.

• 20 million people in the UK are affected by allergies.

See www.immogenics.com, or telephone 0845 226 58 58.

It is important to note that many people cut out hundreds of foodstuffs and become even more sensitive to foods. My experience has been that when the body does show up multiple sensitivities, then emotional stress, lack of sleep, non-absorption, overabundance of chemical products on the body, smoking, alcohol and drug taking are often responsible.

Sometimes the body reacts adversely when deprived of foods it is used to having, so don't worry if you feel unwell for a few days. Whatever your reaction, try to take life quietly and make sure that you don't replace 'forbidden' foods with other bad choices. The list on www.lifesmart.co.uk will show you how to replace forbidden foods with something you are allowed to eat in some of your favourite everyday recipes. Most of the replacement foods are available in health shops and some supermarkets or shops catering for vegetarians, as well as Indian and Chinese supermarkets. Be adventurous with your cooking and, above all, don't feel deprived. Enjoy the new foods and let your friends try your culinary experiments – they may even offer more suggestions.

You can also visit www.lifesmart.co.uk to see a list of common allergens which your GP or complementary practitioner can test for. Their methods of testing may vary. Some are far more accurate than others, but the benefits of knowing your sensitivities is unquestionable. Don't hesitate to get a second opinion if you're not sure about the results. Equally you can ask a nutritionist to help guide you on your own elimination programme of testing food.

Good Cooking Methods

Once you've bought the right foods, it is vitally important to know how to cook and prepare them properly. Some cooking processes can actually produce toxins that weren't there before – specifically browning and burning foods, resulting in known free-radical carcinogens. The skill in cooking well is to produce flavourful, healthy and attractive food with the minimum loss of nutrients. During the cooking process vitamins, minerals, enzymes and other nutrients are to a significant extent destroyed. That's why even when buying high-quality, fresh food, we may not get as many vitamins and minerals as we think.

The vitamins that dissolve in water, such as vitamin C and the B vitamins, are especially vulnerable because they are sensitive to heat and can leach out into the cooking water when they're soaked, blanched or boiled. For example, when cabbage is put in cold water and brought to the boil, it loses 75 per cent of its vitamin content. Fresh peas boiled for five minutes lose 20–40 per cent of their thiamine (a B-vitamin); if lettuce is soaked in water for too long much of its folic acid is lost; and salad vegetables left in water for more than 15 minutes lose 30 per cent of their vitamin C content.

A full breakdown can be found at www.lifesmart.co.uk.

Taking Supplements

When it comes to the design of most nutritional supplements, often the chemistry of what is required to actually make them 'work' in the body is incorrect.

The most basic building block of our bodies is the cell. Approximately every seven years, every cell in our body will have replaced itself. Depending on the organ or body part, some cells do this at a more accelerated rate than others. The most interesting aspect of this 'replacement process' is that the replacement cells are either stronger or weaker than the original depending on environmental factors, genetics, stress and, most importantly, nutrition.

To help our cells move in the direction of life, nature provides us with nutrients. The majority of these nutrients are found in the soil. Minerals, for example calcium, magnesium, boron or zinc, are found as rock particles in the ground. But as the body cannot use nutrients in rock form, nature gave us plants to prepare the nutrients in a way that the body can use. Although this may seem obvious, remember it is only through this natural process that our bodies can best use the nutrients found in the soil. That's why we harvest crops for consumption instead of just consuming 'dirt' with mineral particles in it.

When a plant absorbs a nutrient 'rock' particle from the soil, for example calcium carbonate – a common form of calcium used in supplements today – it begins to work on that particle and put it into a design that is both recognizable and usable by our bodies. The first step is to take that rock and make it soluble. When something enters our body the goal of the digestive process is always the same – liquefaction, or making things soluble. Once this soluble material has entered into the digestive process, the 'soldiers' in our bodies go to work. They 'liberate' the nutrients inside the soluble material and separate them into their respective components. Waste is removed and nutrients are used.

In this 'liberation' process, nutrients, such as minerals, are separated from other components they were once attached to. This is very important. The calcium carbonate rock, for example, is broken down into two parts – $Ca(2+)$ and $CO3(2-)$. However, it is the $Ca(2+)$, or calcium ion, that our cells are able to effectively use as a nutrient for building bone, teeth and tissue. And it is the plant 'preparation process' that allows the 'soldiers' in our bodies to do their work and 'liberate' the nutrients into a design that can be used by the cells in our bodies – a design known as 'cell ready'. This 'cell ready' design also incorporates a correct 'size' of the nutrient molecule. Our cells are very, very small and a nutrient particle cannot be larger than the cell, otherwise it would never get 'in' and be used. Again, it is the plant preparation process that helps to produce a particle size that, once the 'soldiers' in our bodies have 'liberated' the nutrient, can then be used by our cells.

Due to the fact that soils have been significantly depleted of their nutrient content as a result of modern, mass farming techniques, people have turned to supplements for help in satisfying their bodies' nutritional needs. But the key point to understand here is that the design of most nutritional supplements is not the same as the design needed by the body to effectively use nutrients.

Traditional tablets and pills, for example, take mineral rock particles from the soil and crush them up, glue them together and then press them into tablets or pills with a waxy, protective coating. Not only is it hard for the digestive system to 'get past' the waxy coatings and access nutrients inside the tablet, but even worse, since there has been no plant 'preparation process', the 'soldiers' in our bodies cannot effectively use the nutrients.

Using the same example as before, if the 'soldiers' cannot 'liberate' the nutrients, the calcium carbonate remains as calcium carbonate – otherwise known as limestone or blackboard chalk. And so, as with most supplements, the 'soldiers' simply pass the pills and nutrients out of the body – have you ever noticed how the colour of your urine changes when you take supplements?

Because supplement manufacturers have not been able to perfect the plant preparation process characteristics of being water-soluble, ionic and cell ready, some manufacturers have added things to their supplements to help 'encourage' our body's 'soldiers' to liberate the nutrients in their supplements even though the nutrients may not be in the preferred 'plant prepared' design. These types of supplements are often called chelated products.

But what happens if our body's 'soldiers' aren't able to cooperate? Isn't one of the reasons many people supplement because something is already wrong with their bodies? Even if we're healthy, aren't our 'soldiers' busy enough already trying to compensate for synthetic ingredients, strong preservatives, toxins and junk food? For this reason, chelated supplement products also have limited effectiveness.

If you do take supplements, don't be fooled by marketing ploys. Avoid wasting your money on supplements that will not deliver the results you desire and do your research before you buy any supplements. Rotate what you take in order to avoid supplement toxification or immunity, and never think the more you take the better.

Without the presence of necessary minerals to act as co-factors, vitamins are almost worthless anyway, because minerals control the body's ability to absorb and use vitamins. But taking a multi-nutrient pill is not necessarily the answer, as too high a dose of one mineral inhibits the absorption of others.

In other words, whether you need to take dietary supplements – and, if so, which ones – is a complicated issue and it may be advisable to see an expert who can specifically prescribe for your individual needs. It's certainly more complex than just grabbing a bottle off a supermarket shelf as you rush past on the weekly shop. Stress levels, food sensitivities and allergies, genetic make-up, age, gender, activity levels and pollution exposure all determine what each individual needs. As we get older, our bodies absorb less of any vitamins and minerals.

Often a digestive system is so impaired that a capsule or pill form of a supplement may simply aggravate it at first. Also, if this type of supplement is processed too quickly the body does not receive full or lasting benefits. That is why it's so important to know that you have a choice of ways in which you can take a supplement. You can take them through tinctures, loose herbs, in powder, liquid or homeopathic form. Most nutrients can be found in organic loose dried herbs and made up as a tea which is a superb and easy way for the body to absorb it fully. Certain sea vegetables, algaes, grasses, seeds and alfalfa, known as super foods, provide a mix of proteins, vitamins, minerals, antioxidants and trace elements in exactly the right proportions. As they are digested in the same way as foodstuffs, through the bowel and not the urinary system they are highly absorbable and bring numerous benefits including improved digestion, increased alkalinity and greater mental agility and alertness. Wheat and barley also contain antioxidant enzymes that protect healthy cells and guard against the detrimental effects of environmental pollution and stress.

Chlorella is superb for eliminating gut parasites, while algae and spirulina are excellent for building the alkalinity in the body and are good alternatives to multivitamins. Spirulina is rich in vitamin B12, vitamin E, beta-carotene, vitamin C, organic iron, chlorophyll and protein, and is excellent for vegetarians or anyone who feels they need extra supplementation. There are some people who find it particularly hard to assimilate green foods and are probably better off having a powdered form of a multivitamin. Homeopathic tissue salts (of which there are 12) are based on essential minerals that dissolve on the tongue and are also worth exploring. These work particularly well with good nutrition as they help to carry nutrients into the cell. Enviva is a groundbreaking company that has devised cellular friendly supplements. See www.lifesmart.co.uk.

Natural supplements that I have found useful include:
• Flax seed oil. This is the most complete oil to take as it contains all the omega components that the body needs to maintain good health.
• Acidophilus and bifidus probiotics. These counteract the effects of antibiotics and re-establish the presence of beneficial flora in the intestinal tract.
• Aloe vera juice. This is good for cleansing, healing and helping digestive trouble. However, it can be abused so use it sparingly.

Tissue Salts

Usually when my body goes haywire I visit my mentor, Elizabeth Gibaud. Nine times out of 10 there will be two or three tissue salts that I am lacking in, and within 36 hours of replacing these salts I feel completely different. The human body contains 12 vital inorganic elements which are responsible for the maintenance of normal cell function. When one or more of these elements become deficient the normal cell function or metabolism is disturbed. By supplying the lacking elements in the form of tissue salts, normal cell function and health can be restored.

Colloidal Silver

Colloidal minerals are derived from prehistoric plant life. First discovered in the US on a Utah mountaintop 70 years ago, colloidals are microscopic-sized electrically charged particles. When absorbed by the body they act as a magnet, eliminating broken-down cells from the bloodstream. They are an excellent source of plant-derived mineral supplementation and can also be used to treat infections that may arise throughout the body, as well as colds and flu. You can take them in spray or drop form and Sovereign Silver is, I think, one of the best makes available.

See www.lifesmart.co.uk for a guide to useful supplements at various stages in life. See www.sovereign.info for colloidal silver.

Foods To Cut Down On Or Avoid

This section will explain why so many nutritionists, regimes and books advise you to cut out or reduce your intake of the following foodstuffs. Before you panic, you are not being advised to cut anything out for ever. Once you are in good shape and have achieved your health and weight-loss goals, you will know exactly what foods you can include back into your diet.

By cutting down on certain foodstuffs you can discourage unhealthy fluids and toxins from building up in your system, which may cause the following symptoms: cellulite spots; congested bowels; arthritis; bad breath; bleeding gums; low energy; thrush; cystitis and bladder problems; candida; period pains; ME (Myalgic Encephalomyelitis); headaches; body odour; stomach disorders; allergies; tension; irritation and depression; indigestion; ulcers; bad circulation; excess weight; PMS; yellowing eye-whites; back ache; nervousness; discoloured skin; sleeplessness; skin disorders; recurring colds and flu and many more.

Salt

Sodium chloride (salt) is essential for life as it maintains the equilibrium between fluids in the body. Salt also regulates the acid balance and works with potassium to optimize muscle contractions, nerve transmissions and carbon dioxide transportation. Unfortunately, we have tipped the scales with the use of additives and preservatives in processed foods, for example monosodium glutamate (MSG) in meats, stock cubes etc. Primitive man consumed large amounts of vegetable potassium which kept sodium levels balanced. Now we consume far more sodium and far less potassium.

The amount of salt eaten in an average diet has become detrimental. On the reactive side excess salt creates water retention which immediately affects the kidneys' work in balancing the body's water. This can exacerbate pre-menstrual tension as well as causing your system to become constipated, building up toxic fluids which can result in anything from cellulite to more serious problems. All this decreases the body's ability to digest food and to retain vital minerals such as calcium. It also increases cholesterol and can cause weight gain. Sugar cravings commonly occur as a result of having too much salt.

It's actually the sodium part of the salt that is important as sodium, which is the key element in the blood and the fluid surrounding the cells, takes water with it wherever it goes. Our bodies need approximately 500 to1000 mg of salt per day. This is less than a teaspoon and can be handled easily when we eat fresh, natural foods throughout the day. Nowadays processed foods remove much of the natural salts and then manufacturers add more salt and often white sugar for extra flavour. Without us knowing it we become quite addicted to that taste – from babyfoods up – and then we have the seesaw of craving both sugar and salt in equal measure. Salt is also one of the causes of high blood pressure.

Table salt is often refined through heat processing and is bleached with chemicals to make it evenly white. Another chemical, aluminium stearate, is then added so that the salt flows well and doesn't clump. (Natural salts will stick together when they become moist.)

Try not having salt for two weeks and see how bitter food tastes when you add it in again. The cleanest salt both for eating and using medicinally as a gargle for throat infections and as a toxin eliminator in the bath is Himalayan crystal salt from Bestcare Products (see page 205).

Chemicals such as monosodium glutamate, which is commonly used in Chinese cooking; sodium nitrate, a carcinogen used to preserve cured meats; and aspartame are good examples of what needs to be eliminated from your diet. Packaged, processed, pre-cooked shop-bought stock cubes, ready-made cakes, tarts, tinned foods, in other words practically anything that isn't fresh, organic or biodynamic will contain detrimental ingredients. If you don't believe me, do your usual shop, and before you pay for the food put to one side anything that isn't free of MSG, sodium nitrate or aspartame.

Sugar

White sugar and supermarket brown sugar have no fibre content. White sugar is especially bad as it is a refined carbohydrate and the chemical processes involved in turning a naturally brown substance into a snow white powder entail the use of bleaches and other agents. All of these have a detrimental effect on our system, from the intestinal tract to the colon. As a result, it is damaging to the intestinal bacteria and mineral status. This affects the blood content, which in turn affects the brain and causes reactions throughout the body. It exhausts the pancreas and the adrenal glands, causing reactive hypoglycaemia. For example, some hyperactivity and destructive behaviour in children is thought to result from excess sugar intake; similar mental effects, causing altered behaviour and thought patterns can be observed in adults.

The following conditions can be strongly associated with significant sugar consumption: obesity; diabetes mellitus (adult type); gastrointestinal disease (indigestion, inflammatory bowel diseases, irritable bowel syndrome, diarrhoea); gallstones; tooth decay; kidney stones; skin disorders; constant mucus membrane problems (colds, flu, headaches).

Remember that in many forms sugar is toxic, so always read food labels. The less sugar you have the better so that when you do ingest it your body will have no adverse reactions. In some cases honey or fructose sugar may be used sparingly, but no more than two teaspoons in any one serving. Sugar is as potent as any drug and negatively affects the body and the brain. I strongly recommend you buy the book *Sugar Blues* by William Dufty to discover more.

The main foods containing sugar that should be avoided, or cut down to once a week at most, are: malt; some mustards; cakes and pies; some vinegars; tinned foods; molasses; biscuits; most breads; all alcohol; ketchup; bottled sauces; packaged muesli; glucose; mayonnaise; ready-made meals.

For the serious sugar addict, or people who are very allergic or sensitive to sugar, you may also have to cut out: maple syrup; figs; dried fruits; honey; raisins; dates; grapes.

Just about every pre-prepared, bottled or packaged food contains sugar. Beware also of some tropical fruits, which are toxic to those with sugar allergies.

Sugar is the most common addiction of all. Too much sugar is associated with heart disease, diabetes, tooth decay and obesity. Frequent overuse of sugar can lead to what is known as glucose intolerance, which means an abnormal blood sugar balance. The symptoms may include irritability, aggressive outbursts, nervousness, depression, crying spells, dizziness, fears and anxiety, confusion, forgetfulness, inability to concentrate, fatigue, insomnia, headaches, palpitations, muscle cramps, excess sweating, digestive problems, allergies, blurred vision, excessive thirst and a lack of sex drive. Does this sound like anyone you know? Probably seven in every 10 people have a mild form of blood sugar imbalance.

• Over 2.5 million people in the UK are living with heart disease, and each year around 250,000 people die from it.

We all have a natural sweet tooth, but the more sweet foods we eat, the greater our taste for sweetness. In nature, sweet foods are uncommon and are usually safe to eat. But by refining sugar we've learnt how to cheat nature and eat sugar in a pure form. Nowadays, concentrated sugar comes in many guises – glucose, dextrose, maltose, honey and syrups among others. All these help to develop a sweet tooth, as does any food with concentrated sweetness, including grape juice or too much dried fruit such as raisins, although the sugar in most fruit (fructose) does not have the same effect on the body as glucose, maltose or sucrose (normal sugar). They do, however, cause fermentation and the amount you eat has to be regulated.

Often people think that fructose is a totally acceptable alternative to sugar and that it won't lead to weight gain because it is a natural fruit sugar – but the only way that fructose is acceptable is when it comes with the fruit itself, which contains fibre and other nutrients to slow down the release of the fructose. High-fructose corn syrup has recently been developed as a cheaper, longer-life sugar alternative – eight times sweeter than refined sugar and highly resistant to bacteria, it is easier to blend into drinks and foods. British imports of this sweetener have increased nearly seven fold from 5,000 tonnes to almost 34,000 in the past four years. This is just one example of the many unwanted and unnecessary ingredients put into an array of convenience and junk foods and drinks, which as an ordinary consumer we don't bother to think about. We just get hooked, fat and more unwell.

Kicking the sugar habit takes time and perseverance. It is best to wean yourself off slowly so that your taste buds get used to less and less sweetness. Stop adding sugar to cereals and eating cereals containing sugar, use aguave syrup and a small amount of honey or maple syrup instead until you feel you don't need to sweeten your cereal. When you want something sweet have a piece of fresh fruit – as long as it's a couple of hours before or after a meal so that you don't interrupt your digestion and elimination process. Get used to diluting fruit juices with water. Gradually decrease your overall intake of sweet foods. Once you're basically sugar-free the odd sweet food is not a problem.

Chocolate

The UK has become one of the largest chocolate and sweet eating nations in the world. We spend billions of pounds on confectionary. Chocolate is full of sugar. It also contains cocoa as its major active ingredient, which provides significant quantities of the stimulant theobromine, whose action is similar to – although not as strong as – caffeine's. Theobromine is also obtained from cocoa drinks such as hot chocolate. Because of the high sugar and stimulant content of chocolate, plus its delicious taste, it's easy to become a chocaholic.

The best way to quit the chocolate habit is to find good alternatives, for example in health food shops. Although these 'alternatives' are ways to wean you off sweets and chocolate, they should be eaten as an occasional treat, not on a daily basis. Be aware also that many so-called health bars are packed with sugar, hydrogenated fat and other not so healthy ingredients – always check the label.

White Flour

Another refined carbohydrate, white flour has no nutritional value as it has been bleached, pumped full of additives and preservatives (which many of us are allergic to) and has also had all the fibre removed. White flour (and sugar) also create the same effect as an alcoholic reaction in the body, hence why many addiction counsellors suggest their clients avoid this.

Wheat

Wheat is such a common food that we find it hard to imagine that it might be the cause of many health problems. In its unrefined state, wheat is a good source of complex carbohydrates, fibre and other nutrients. Yet many people suffer from intolerance to wheat and its byproducts and experience an improvement in their health if they reduce or eliminate wheat from their diet. If you feel below-par it is certainly worth trying. Today's wheat is highly processed and a large proportion of the vitamins, minerals and trace elements are destroyed during the processing.

Why do these problems occur? Three components of the wheat grain can cause trouble: wheat bran, gluten and phytates. Wheat bran is abrasive to the digestive tract and can cause irritation and inflammation.

Gluten, a sticky substance that sticks to the walls of the intestines, makes digestion very difficult and prevents the absorption of nutrients. Did you know that the glue for papier mâché is made of flour and water? Just imagine what bread can do to your digestive tract!

Modern wheat is grown to be especially high in gluten as this protein, in combination with yeast and sugar, helps make bigger and lighter loaves of bread. Grains containing gluten can also be found in rye, oats, spelt and barley. Although these grains do not contain as high a level of gluten as wheat does, they may have to be avoided in severe intolerance cases. If there is no problem with intolerances then they can make an excellent alternative to wheat.

A further problem with wheat is its high phytate content. Phytates are found in the fibre of wheat (and other grains). These substances bind with minerals such as calcium, iron, zinc and copper and inhibit their absorption. Wheat contains a higher level of phytates than many other grains. A bowl of cereal with milk therefore does not provide much calcium as the calcium binds with the phytates and becomes unabsorbable.

Phytates are broken down during the leavening process, so they are more commonly found in breakfast cereals where yeast is not used. Our modern diet already tends to be low in minerals such as iron, zinc and magnesium, due to eating refined foods and to reduced mineral content in the soil, so we do not need to make matters worse by eating an excess of wheat.

Common symptoms associated with wheat intolerance are: constipation; diarrhoea; bloating and discomfort; joint pain; allergies; eczema; asthma; lethargy or sluggishness; digestive problems such as irritable bowel syndrome and water retention; inability to lose weight; nausea; skin rashes; cramps; acne; flatulence; migraines; depression; sweating and anxiety; loss of concentration; rheumatoid arthritis; joint and muscle aches and pains; premenstrual syndrome; chronic fatigue; tissue swelling and coeliac disease.

If you suffer from any of these symptoms it is worth taking a good look at your wheat intake and considering an exploratory exclusion diet. Many people eat wheat three or more times a day, every day. Toast for breakfast, a sandwich for lunch, pasta for dinner, pizza, pastries, cakes, biscuits… eating too much of any one food is never a good idea, and is a certain way of lowering your tolerance to that food.

Wheat-based products include: bread, pasta, sorrel, nut roasts, pastry, bottled sauces (including soy and tamari sauces), cakes, biscuits, batter, crisp breads, muesli, taramasalata, tofu burgers and breakfast cereals. Other wheat sources include bulgur wheat, couscous, durum wheat, faro, kamut, semolina and triticum.

Unless otherwise labelled, wheat-based products also include: bagels, bran, chapattis, crisp bread, crumpets, flour, naan bread, pastry, pitta bread, pizza, pasta, noodles and rusks.

Many ready-made meals and processed foods may also contain wheat. This may be listed as: baking powder, cereal binder, cereal filler, cereal protein, cereal starch, edible starch, food starch, hydrolysed protein, hydrolysed vegetable protein, modified starch, malted flakes, textured vegetable protein, vegetable protein or wheat starch. Thickeners and stabilizers sometimes contain traces of wheat. Note that buckwheat is not actually wheat at all and is therefore a good alternative to wheat, as are quinoa and millet.

If you think you might be intolerant to wheat then try excluding it completely from your diet for six to eight weeks, but do not do this without planning ahead. Seek out alternatives and stock up on them. Think about lunches and plan ahead if you are going to have to buy food out. The first thing you need to know is which foods contain wheat, and then find out which foods you can have instead. It is always important to replace foods that you remove from your diet, and there are many alternatives to wheat-based foods.

After the exclusion period try a reintroduction and pulse test. Prepare a meal with a large amount of wheat in it (more than usual). Relax for five minutes and record your resting pulse rate. Eat the meal and enjoy it! Take your pulse again and record the rate 10 minutes after the meal, then 30 minutes later and finally 60 minutes later. Pay attention to any symptoms over the next day or two and note those down too. If your pulse rose by 10 points or more and/or you experienced symptoms linked to wheat intolerance you may benefit from minimizing or avoiding wheat for the time being.

If you are intolerant to wheat it is not a life sentence. Having wheat on occasion and balancing it in your diet with other grains is the key to enjoying wheat and not letting it hinder your health.

See www.lifesmart.co.uk for a list of alternative non-wheat food products.

Yeast

Ingesting yeast regularly should be avoided because as soon as it comes into contact with other foods containing sugar it begins to ferment, creating gases in the stomach. It is also a contributing factor in the development of thrush, candida, ME and various allergies. It interferes with the bowel flora in the colon, setting up the ideal conditions for unhealthy bacteria to overcome healthy bacteria. As bowel flora is designed to complete the digestive process and control infection from harmful bacteria, viruses, fungi and yeast-eating worms this can cause many problems.

Processed, unnatural foods lacking in fibre, meat contaminated with hormones and antibiotics, vegetables contaminated by fertilizers and pesticides, and faddy diets all create conditions for organisms living on putrefaction.

Antibiotics wipe out the good bacteria (such as lactobacillus) as well as the bad. So *candida albicans*, normally kept in check by good bacteria, is allowed to flourish, spreading to affect the mucus membranes which leads to thrush, respiratory illness, stomach and intestinal irritation and, as a result, allergies and a weak immune system. Yeast intolerance can make a person feel continually unwell and trigger off internal problems such as bloating and stomach cramps.

Yeast is found in some foods or is created in your body as a result of foodstuffs such as dried fruits and alcohol. Foods containing yeast include: alcohol, bread, soy sauce, vinegar, marmite, bouillon, pates (including vegetable pâtés), stock cubes, yeast extract, biscuits, nut roasts and savoury spreads.

Coeliac Disease

Sufferers of coeliac disease are sensitive to a protein found in wheat, spelt, rye, oats and barley. As a result, damage occurs to the lining of the small bowel, which then cannot absorb nutrients. Weight loss, diarrhoea, abdominal bloating, anaemia, fatigue and muscle wasting are just some of the symptoms associated with this problem.

We are seeing a considerable increase of coeliac diease in children, and it is now thought that wheat and other grains introduced too early (they should be avoided for the first year of life) could be a possible contributor. Coeliac disease is also associated with diabetes, infection caused by a virus and thyroid problems amongst other factors. Following a gluten-free diet is essential. Milk products can be another irritant because the lactose present in milk often causes diarrhoea. It's imperative that you are diagnosed by your GP and not just a nutritionist.

See www.lifesmart.co.uk for a list of alternative non-yeast food products.

Dairy Products

If you are intolerant to dairy products then it is advised that dairy products from cows be excluded from your diet completely at first (unless otherwise instructed), and kept to a maximum of twice a week after you have cleared your system. When you introduce dairy products back into your diet stick to organic goat's and sheep's produce.

Although new mothers, babies and infants have a particular need for calcium, remember that calcium is available from a number of healthy non-dairy sources.

Babies should when possible drink their mother's breastmilk – which is considerably different to cow's milk – and contains antibodies and hundreds of nutrients which dairy milk cannot provide.

We have been brainwashed into thinking that dairy products and milk in particular are the only source of calcium. Women especially are often concerned about their calcium intake in order to prevent osteoporosis. However, there are many dairy-free foods that contain high levels of calcium and which can be utilized far more efficiently by the body.

Alternative sources of calcium are now widely available and include: beans, pulses; dark green vegetables (especially broccoli, watercress and parsley); turnips; sesame seeds; almonds; salmon; tofu; and soup (made with stock from bones and one teaspoon of cider vinegar, which draws out the calcium).

Absorption Of Calcium

It is important to realize that you do not only need to eat foods that are high in calcium, but also that the combination of certain foods will affect the absorption of calcium. Substances such as sugar affect calcium absorption, as do high-protein foods, vegetables in the nightshade family, wine, vinegar, citrus fruits, caffeine, alcohol and salt.

Phosphorus must also be present in the diet (dairy food has very little) otherwise calcium passes straight through the system. Phosphorous is found in kelp, rice, sunflower and pumpkin seeds, Brazil nuts, fish, radishes, leeks, prunes, spinach and watercress.

How Different Foods Affect Calcium Absorption

• Concentrated sugars create an acidic reaction which de-mineralizes the system and causes phosphorus levels to drop.
• High-protein foods acidify the blood which dissolves calcium from the bones.
• Plants in the nightshade family – these include tobacco, peppers and tomatoes – neutralize the calcium content in the blood.
• Over-use of highly acidic food and drink such as wine, vinegar, oranges and grapefruits can use up calcium during metabolism. This calcium will be taken from the teeth and bones.
• Caffeine, alcohol and salt all bring about calcium loss and can cause calcium to be excreted instead of being absorbed.

Although dairy produce has a a high calcium content, this calcium is not easily absorbed by the body, leading to several health problems. The adult body needs lactase (an enzyme) to break down and digest the lactose (milk sugars). The ability to produce lactase is not present in some adults and they can become lactose intolerant. The symptoms of lactose intolerance include: digestive discomfort; bloating; wind; irritable bowel syndrome and excessive mucus production.

How Milk Can Affect The Body

Sodium and potassium levels are disrupted by milk intake, which contributes to oedema (water retention) and mineral imbalances.

When milk is pasteurized the good bacteria and enzymes are destroyed. This makes the proteins difficult to digest, and the calcium becomes insoluble.

When milk is combined with wheat a sticky substance is produced, this then clings to the intestines and prevents nutrients from being absorbed. It also creates ideal conditions for the development and growth of putrefying bacteria, leading to problems such as candida and thrush.

The high cholesterol content of dairy products also contributes to the hardening of the arteries. The circulation becomes sluggish and people suffer from excessive tiredness, chest pains and leg cramps. Eventually the arteries may close up altogether leading to heart attacks.

The high fat content of dairy products causes the over-production of oestrogen, leading to a hormonal imbalance. This has been linked not only to breast cancer but also early onset of menstruation in puberty, heavy menstrual flow and late menopause. High fat levels also contribute to weight problems and related symptoms. While low-fat products help to reduce total fat consumption, they nevertheless cause the same problems and symptoms as full-fat versions.

Further symptoms that can be caused or aggravated by dairy products include asthma; bronchitis; hayfever; tonsillitis; a congested lymphatic system; recurring colds; eczema; acne; lethargy; headaches; irritability; menstrual cramps; chronic fatigue and hyperactivity.

Also to be taken into consideration are the modern farming techniques used in dairy farming. Drug treatments including steroids and antibiotics are regularly injected into dairy herds to stimulate extra production of milk. The use of animal feeds containing artificial proteins and pesticides is also a commonplace practice. The effects of these farming practices are only now becoming more widely known.

Ingredients To Watch Out For

Milk and milk products are present in many foods and you will need to familiarize yourself with product labels and the more obscure terminology used when milk is in a product. The most common foods to avoid are: milk, milk powder, butter, milk drinks, cheese, yoghurt, cream, dairy ice cream (in fact all types of dairy). However, it's not always quite so obvious. For example, food labels that list any of the ingredients below also contain some cow's milk or products: casein, caseinates, hydrolysed casein, skimmed milk whey, skimmed milk powder, milk solids, non-fat milk solids, whey syrup sweetener, milk sugar, lactose, whey and ghee.

The following are examples of processed foods which may contain milk: breakfast cereals, soups, baby foods, processed meats such as sliced meats and sausages, pasta, pizzas, instant mashed potato, sauces, gravies, baked goods such as rolls, pancakes, batters, ready-made meals, puddings, custard and chocolate. This lists just some of the foods to be avoided in a dairy-free diet. To be on the safe side, it is always best to read the food labels or check with the retailer.

Non-dairy products are widely available, such as organic soya milk, oat milk, rice milk, soya crème and goat's and sheep's cream and milk. There are also several alternative non-dairy yoghurts, spreads and cheeses.

Soya Bean Milk

This is the heaviest form of vegetable protein to digest (try Bonsoy soya milk first as it is the easiest kind to digest). Use in moderation on cereal or in drinks in place of ordinary cow's milk, but don't use it when making desserts like rice pudding as it uses up too much soya milk (instead use rice or oat milk). It is stocked in good health shops, but do not buy soya milk containing salt or sugar.

See www.lifesmart.co.uk for a list of alternative non-dairy food products.

Meat

Meat is by no means to be avoided, however it is important to be aware of the following. Almost all commercially reared animals in this country have steroids (for artificial increased growth) and antibiotics mixed into their feed. Most of us are allergic to these additives in the short term, and nobody quite knows what they will do to us when eaten in large amounts, or more than twice a week, in the long term.

Red meat can also place a burden on our system as it requires a great deal of energy to break it down into amino acids. Also, if the kidneys find it difficult to excrete all the toxins that red meat produces, they may accumulate in the tissues and joints, crystallize and cause considerable health problems. Large quantities of protein can overwhelm the system which leads to partly digested peptide molecules; because they are left undigested in the colon, toxins form and putrefaction develops, causing allergic reactions.

Red meat also tends to be high in fat. For instance, a slice of ham is 25 per cent protein and 75 per cent fat, while a plate of beans is 36 per cent protein and just six per cent fat.

Processed Food

Avoid processed food! The preservatives, colourings, salt, sugar, cheap fats and cheap ingredients used in processed and fast foods have no nutritional value and are bad for us. Without additives and preservatives the foods would spoil very quickly. The fact that food goes stale in its natural state is for our own protection – it begins to look and taste unappetizing so we won't eat it. Just consider the number of chemicals added to foods to maintain their appearance from the time they leave the factory until the time they arrive on your plate. Smoked meats and fish contain high quantities of sodium nitrate and when these are combined with other chemicals in the stomach they produce nitrosamines. Nitrosamines are the most potent cancer-producing substances which have so far been discovered by scientists.

Processing and cooking foods – especially at high temperatures – alter the food's fat, protein and fibre content, and also destroy many of the essential nutrients. The body recognizes cooked and processed foods and views them as harmful invaders, so it does its best to eradicate them. Simply put, white blood cells rush to the intestines as soon as food enters the mouth – this doesn't happen when raw foods are eaten – and this process leaves the rest of the body undefended, placing a huge strain on the immune system. Raw foods leave the white blood cells free and the body is saved the effort of evasive action, thereby strengthening its resistance to disease.

Fried foods are especially bad. The oil used for frying is generally of poor quality and, at high temperatures, is damaged by oxygen, turning it into a toxin that is harmful to the body. Fried foods also line the digestive tract causing indigestion, bowel congestion, a bad taste in the mouth and bad breath – quite apart from the fact that it has little nutritional value and can lead to more serious illnesses.

Curries And Highly Spiced Foods

Mild spices are generally accepted by the digestive system and the body. However, high-voltage curries and other spiced foods are not. Consider how you feel after a hot curry, with a flushed face and perspiring body and you'll have an idea of what is going on inside you. Your digestive system is in violent uproar, trying to cope with the onslaught. If you must eat curry and hot spices, drink plenty of water to help the body cope and flush away the toxins.

Eggs

Eggs are commonly known to have a negative effect on childhood disorders, including eczema, hyperactivity, sleep disturbances and behavioural disorders. Egg yolk is high in cholesterol and should therefore not be eaten in excess (although it is rich in vitamins and minerals), but egg whites are a good source of protein. Eggs suffer the indignities of commercial production as much as chickens (antibiotics, chemical feed and hormones) – so buy organic or free-range eggs and eat no more than four a week. Some people are sensitive to egg yolk, but not white, although often eggs cooked in food (such as cakes), will not produce an allergic reaction in an egg-sensitive person.

• Eczema has increased 300 per cent in the past 30 years. One in five children and one in 12 adults now suffer from it.

The Nightshade Family And Other 'Stressful' Vegetables

The nightshade family, which includes tomatoes, potatoes, aubergine and peppers, is one group of vegetables that you should eat in moderation, especially in times of stress. Studies have shown that they speed up the heart rate and slow down digestion. They are high in alkaloids which block B vitamin absorption (a key vitamin for coping with stress) and may contribute to arthritic and rheumatic symptoms.

Other vegetables that can be irritating to our bodies include shard, spinach, beets and rhubarb. These contain oxalic acid which binds calcium and eliminates it from the body. This is seen as a possible risk of osteoporosis and kidney stones.

No one is saying that you should cut these foods out of your diet completely or that they are wholly bad, as in fact they all have excellent properties. You just need to be aware that they can cause problems.

Nuts

Nuts, as well as being a common allergen, are very hard to digest and should not be eaten unless your bowels and digestive system, weight, skin and circulation are working to perfection.

All About Liquids

Water is the beginning and end of all life forms. Our health and that of this planet is dependent upon it. Seventy per cent of the planet is covered in water and 70 per cent of our body is made up of water. It penetrates every cell and regulates all bodily functions. Water cleanses the body, transports nutrients, removes waste and regulates our body temperature. On a daily basis our bodies discharge approximately two to two-and-a-half litres of water, and this constant loss of fluid needs to be constantly replenished.

Knowing all this, I find it incredible how many people don't know about the importance of drinking plain water. These days, people don't think twice about drinking liquids and so-called energy drinks that are high in caffeine, sugar, acidic fruit sugar, preservatives, acids, salt and gas. Many people are mistaken in the assumption that all fluids are equivalent to water. But these drinks are in part contributing to our ill health and weight problems. Our choice of fluid is more likely to disturb the whole digestive system and actually have a toxic and diuretic, or dehydrating effect, on the body than what we eat. The toxins from these drinks infiltrate the bloodstream, which in turn can affect your skin, blood sugar levels and gastric health.

Learning how to flush and hydrate the body properly is one of the most important changes any one of us can make. This helps prevent a build-up of rubbish and allows metabolism to occur at its natural rate. Try drinking only pure, uncarbonated water for one week and see what a difference it makes to symptoms such as fatigue, headaches, blotchy skin, brittle bones, arthritis and dark circles under the eyes.

When we are dehydrated the body conserves and rations the water available to it. Urine and sweat production are reduced and more water is extracted from the contents of the colon (a common cause of constipation). By not drinking enough water, we become less able to eliminate poisonous waste products, resulting in headaches, lethargy and bad breath. More importantly, it's the beginning of a slow decline in the body as a whole. Another response the body makes to dehydration is to increase the production of cholesterol. This is incorporated into the membranes surrounding the body cells so that they become less permeable, a protective move by the body to avoid fluid losses from inside the cells. But it also means that nutrients are less able to enter the cells and toxins cannot escape, which leads to stagnation.

A further consequence of dehydration is that water is rationed and reserved for the most essential functions at the expense of less urgent needs. One of the first functions to suffer is the removal of cellular waste via the lymphatic system and the body becomes sluggish and smelly. Most of us are therefore unable to blossom to our full potential due to lack of water.

Water – When And How

One of the biggest mistakes that people make, even if they drink their required amount of water in a given day, is to have juice or a cup of tea or coffee as their first drink of the day. This is a problem because at night toxins rise to the surface and they need to be flushed out of your body by water first thing. Drinking water will also help your body cope with any imbalance or cravings due to any foods you may have eaten the night before.

You should drink water between sunrise and sunset, aiming to drink on average one-and-a-half to two-and-a-half litres every day. Drink still, bottled water as carbonated water has too much sodium (salt) and may upset the stomach as well as causing burping and flatulence. Tap water (apart from tasting foul), is recycled many times in England and even filtering is not enough to eliminate all the hormones from the urine of women who are taking the Pill or HRT.

Water should be drunk at room temperature – cold or iced water shocks the system and can cause stomach aches and interfere with digestion. Water flushes the kidneys and washes the bladder, cleaning away acidity and infection. Medically, it literally washes away impurities, regulates the concentration of salts and the acid balance of the blood, thereby excreting all waste products. Lack of water causes the kidneys stress – they need a constant supply to function effectively and keep the bladder clean, fresh and comfortable.

As your body slows down during the evening, the main organs, including the liver and kidneys, 'change gear' and perform different functions to those carried out during the day. The body is programmed to heal and recuperate throughout the night and so the body slows down. The kidneys begin processing fluids differently, focusing on breaking down stored poisons from the day.

It is important to start drinking water when you get up, and to have a steady intake all day long so that you don't end up being dehydrated at night time. Many people make the mistake of drinking their quota of water during the night, which puts undue pressure on their system.

After 6pm it is therefore best to drink herbal teas or water with a squeeze of lemon or lime. However, make sure you keep your intake to a minimum as the body doesn't like to hold large amounts of liquid at night – try not to drink for at least two hours before you go to bed.

Drinking And Eating

Don't drink half an hour before, during, or half an hour to an hour after a meal as it dilutes all the digestive enzymes, allowing food to 'swim' around becoming more toxic rather than being digested unhindered. Many nutrients get lost and your energy levels will plummet. Flatulence, indigestion, water retention, headaches and bad breath may be problems. A tiny amount of pure, flat water, vegetable juice or good-quality wine is fine if sipped, but check your gastric reaction – if any gas forms or you get indigestion it's best avoided. If you get really thirsty (enough to want to gulp down a lot of liquid), you're using unnecessary amounts of spices or salt in seasonings, or mixing too much sweet and sour. Try chewing on cucumber after a meal, then brush your teeth – this should remove thirst-inducing items from your mouth. If you are still feeling thirsty, sipping fresh mint tea should suffice. If you feel bloated or sick after a meal, drink a cup of hot water with celery leaves seeped in it – it's a wonderful cleanser. A glass of water with a teaspoon of organic cider vinegar is also excellent if you have any sort of stomach problem or headache.

Coffee

I know everyone loves coffee. Interestingly, nine out of 10 people, when asked what their first recollection of tasting coffee was, replied that they turned their nose up and at best thought it tasted bitter. Coffee is very similar to a Turkish sweet called Halva, and the reaction at first is the same as caffeine – once tried, you've just got to have more. Before you know it, you are completely addicted. Most of us weren't brought up to drink plenty of water to replenish our energy levels, nor to enjoy hot water with either lemon, ginger, fresh mint or other herbal choices. Remember: these hot drinks increase your energy levels just by hydrating your system while being both refreshing and uplifting, without containing stimulants. Yet coffee and tea remain the drink of the day, and unfortunately to our detriment. A really delicious fresh cup of coffee once in a while and when you are relaxed or on holiday is absolutely fine, but the present-day drip-feed of coffee is depleting you physically and mentally.

Coffee contains three stimulants – caffeine, theobromine and theophylline – all of which are addictive. Although caffeine is the strongest, theobromine has a similar effect, it is just present in much smaller amounts. Theophylline is known to disturb normal sleep patterns. Decaffeinated coffee still provides theophylline and theobromine so it isn't stimulant-free.

People who consume a lot of coffee have a greater risk of a variety of health problems and a higher incidence of birth defects in their children. Coffee stops vital minerals from being absorbed, for example the amount of iron absorbed from food is reduced by two-thirds if coffee is drunk with a meal.

If you stop drinking coffee, you may get withdrawal symptoms for up to three days, which reflects how addicted you've become. After that, if you begin to feel perky and your health improves it's a good indication that you're better off without coffee. The most popular alternatives to coffee are Caro Extra (made with roasted barley, chicory and rye); Barley Cup; dandelion coffee (Symingtons or Lanes) or herb teas. Also check your health food shop for new coffee substitutes.

Tea

Tea is the great British addiction. A strong cup of tea contains as much caffeine as a weak cup of coffee and is certainly addictive. Tea also contains tannin, which interferes with the absorption of vital minerals such as iron and zinc. Like coffee, drinking too much tea is associated with a number of health problems including an increased risk of stomach ulcers. Particularly addictive is Earl Grey tea, which contains bergamot, itself a stimulant.

The best-tasting alternatives to regular tea are peppermint, fennel, green and fruit teas. Drinking very weak (regular) tea occasionally is unlikely to be a problem, but if you drink tea, make sure it's a really good-quality, organic brand without the chemicals and additives that are found in the cheaper brands.

See www.lifesmart.co.uk for a list of alternatives.

Carbonated Drinks

Cola and some other fizzy drinks contain between five and seven milligrams of caffeine – roughly a quarter of that found in a weak cup of coffee. In addition, these drinks are often high in sugar and colourings and their net stimulant effect can be considerable. Check the ingredients list and stay away from drinks containing caffeine and chemical additives or colourings. Many fizzy drinks also contain phosphoric acid, and once inside the body this acid reaches the bloodstream and lowers the pH. In order to restore the blood to its normal levels, the body looks for an alkaline molecule to counteract the acid – and the easiest one to find is calcium, which it takes from the bones. Finally, the diet drinks may contain chemical sweeteners such as aspartame, which in itself is addictive and has many side effects.

Alcohol

Alcohol is chemically very similar to sugar, and is high in calories. It disturbs normal blood sugar balance and appetite. Enough alcohol suppresses appetite, which leads to more 'empty' calories from alcohol and less nutritious calories from healthy food. Alcohol also destroys or prevents the absorption of many nutrients including vitamin C, the B vitamins, calcium, magnesium and zinc. Best results are achieved in an initial nutritional programme if you cut out alcohol entirely, or have no more than three small drinks each week.

Alcohol is a major irritant to the walls of the intestines and is a specific threat to the liver. Alcohol enters directly into the bloodstream and it remains there for an extended period of time, which makes the sugar it contains extremely difficult to eliminate. The effect of this is to slow down the reactions of the mind and body. Alcohol causes a tendency to have cellulite and broken veins and continual mucus-based problems, for example colds, flu and chest congestion.

Alcohol is thought of as a stimulant but is in fact a brain depressant. Drinking alcohol gives a false sense of self-confidence and ability to communicate, but the real effect of alcohol is that it depresses the function of the brain and its ability to deal with trauma. Too much alcohol has an adverse effect on the metabolic and nutritional state of the body. Obesity is common amongst alcohol consumers, especially young beer drinkers. Women metabolize alcohol at a faster rate than men and therefore feel the effects of alcohol much sooner. Women who drink excessively are also at more risk of developing cirrhosis of the liver.

Sweet wine, champagne, red wine, beer, lager and cider all have a high sugar content and are therefore highly acidic.

If you do drink alcohol, drink it during a meal, no more than once or twice a week and no more than two glasses at one time, so the toxins can be absorbed by the food instead of your nervous system. Try to drink plenty of water with it to flush it through your system. Sip slowly and control the amount you consume.

Organic/biodynamic alcohol does not have any chemicals which could cause extra aggravation. Many people think that alcohol which is organic/biodynamic is not real alcohol or that it will taste awful. On the contrary, even hard-nosed experts will tell you that the taste is superior, plus you won't get the physical reactions that can occur when you drink ordinary wine.

Alcohol Dependency

I am constantly saddened by the enormous number of 'ordinary', 'well-adjusted', 'educated' men and women who have a dependency on alcohol, yet don't even consider this to be the case. They are all such totally different characters yet the self-sabotage is painfully evident. There may be a number of reasons and categories of people:

• One in 15 doctors is addicted to either drugs or alcohol.

1. People who are lonely. They may be missing a spouse who is often away, which means they are not able to relax sufficiently or sleep easily. Ongoing difficulties with children, whether they are energetically a handful or disabled in some way. Unequal sharing of young children due to partner being absent, a workaholic or away all the time.

2. Women who have been unable to have children may throw everything into working and living hard and fast, even if they are happily married. These people are often good at dealing with other people's problems, either at work or socially. They take on the troubles of the world and they use alcohol as their prop – they usually drink too much and allow themselves to lose

control. They normally have a history of this throughout their adult life, either with alcohol, food, smoking or drugs.

3. Married couples with children who are high achievers and workers, and are active in the community, may work and play hard – eating and drinking to excess almost daily. (It is important to note that it is common to see these people smoke cigarettes when they are out, or smoke dope privately indoors, even though they are not everyday smokers.)

4. Students and adults in their twenties whose whole social existence revolves around pubs, bars and wine bars. It is very rare to find a young person who does not drink or smoke, and this is especially common in the major cities. It is not until they start to settle down, perhaps after marriage, that they calm down enough not to need the courage or the stimulation that they feel alcohol gives them. Once in a stable relationship they may no longer need to fill the gap with drinking and socializing in this way, and it is only then that they begin to question and change their habits.

5. Many of the people I have worked with as clients or dealt with in the fashion world, the arts and commerce, especially the high achievers and workaholics, married or otherwise, seem to have a huge need 'to use' alcohol. This usually goes hand in hand with feeling they get a lack of recognition and acknowledgment from their peers, friends and particularly spouses. They often feel unseen or in others' shadows, and drink is rife in these cases. Little of this is ever expressed, and their home lives tend to be chaotic.

6. Another category are men and women who have married very young and where either both parties, or just one, hits an early mid-life crisis; having had two or more children by the age of 30, they are desperate to break out of the confines of their lives but are tied to their obligations. Alcohol as well as recreational drug-taking becomes a means of escape, but it destroys relationships and creates bad role models for the children.

It is truly heartbreaking to see the effect of alcohol in all these different examples, as well as others I haven't mentioned. Especially because, to be an addict people think you have to have several bottles of alcohol a day, wake up and start drinking straight away and so on. *I am sorry to say that this is not the case, not only with alcohol but all forms of fats, sugars, food etc. that people seem to find impossible to cut out of their life.* It is often not until something serious occurs, such as ulcers, newly diagnosed diabetes, or some other health scare, that we consider taking any action.

• Liver disease caused by excessive drinking has reportedly risen by 75 per cent in just six years.

When It's Okay To Drink Alcohol

You know by your own condition whether you can tolerate alcohol or not, but basically do not imbibe alcohol until you have cleaned your system out properly. It takes 30 days to clear out any poisons in the body, including alcohol, and another 30 or more depending on your past intake of alcohol to repair and begin to build up the strength of your immune system. Only then may your system be strong enough to tolerate alcohol again.

Guidelines
1. Drink alcohol with a meal rather than on its own so that the food can act as a cushion and absorb the toxins rather than your nervous system absorbing it all.
2. Sip slowly and don't ever overdose on the amount you have.
3. Make sure you are drinking the very best-quality alcohol that you can, and if possible, try organic/biodynamic wines.
4. Keep your intake to weekends only, rather than using alcohol to relax you on a nightly basis, which doesn't work in the long term as alcohol is a depressant, both emotionally and energetically.

When alcohol is taken in moderation and at the right time it can aid digestion. For example, the liqueurs Strega and Benedictine are the most beneficial kinds of alcohol to have after an evening meal.

Processed Drinks
Squashes, cordials and sports drinks are full of ingredients your body can do without. Remember even though they are liquids and not in a solid form they are just as likely to pile on the pounds and erode the body.

Diet drinks can cause weight gain. Although they contain virtually no calories they are possibly the cause of weight gain because the chemicals that are used in sugar substitutes can create toxic by-products which the liver then packages up in the fat cells. In addition, the sugar substitutes do not alleviate the sugar cravings, and, if anything, make them worse. People become addicted to diet drinks and despite all other efforts continue to gain weight. Eighty-four per cent of all sodas consumed belong to two companies: Coca-Cola have 48.2 per cent of the market and Pepsi-Cola 35.9 per cent. Over 90 per cent of all diet sodas consumed contain caffeine and aspartame.

Caffeine, as already mentioned, is an addictive drug. It also acts on the kidneys and causes increased urine production, dehydrating your body. This characteristic is the main reason why a person is forced to drink so many cans of soda every day yet is never satisfied. The water from the soda does not stay in the body long enough to rehydrate, and most people confuse being hungry with being thirsty. So over time the dehydration caused by caffeine-containing sodas may cause a gradual gain in weight.

In the early 1980s a new product called aspartame was introduced to the beverage industry as an artificial sweetener to replace saccharin. It was 190 times sweeter than sugar without any calorie output and is now in common use because the Food and Drug Administration (FDA) has deemed it safe to use in

• Ten of the UK's biggest-selling soft drinks have been found to contain more than 70 additives, many linked to hyperactivity, asthma, tooth decay, sleep disturbance, diabetes and cancer.

place of sugar. In the intestinal tract, aspartame converts to two highly excitatory neurotransmitter amino acids: phenylalanine and methyl alcohol/ formaldehyde wood alcohol. It is claimed that the liver renders methyl alcohol non-toxic. I personally think this claim is made to brush aside voiced objections for commercialization of a manufactured 'food' that has a known toxic byproduct.

The chemicals added to the sodas are absorbed in the cells of the body and the brain, which upsets your natural chemical balance – the very balance that your body is always striving to maintain. Any ingredients that disturb the natural biological workings of the body will impede proper energy release.

Children in particular become vulnerable to the addictive properties of beverages containing caffeine. Stimulating the body in the early stages of life with pleasure-enhancing chemicals in beverages could establish addictive behaviour in later life.

People who want to continue to consume diet sodas may benefit from reading extensive research available on the internet concerning aspartame and similar chemicals used in these drinks.

Red Bull

Red Bull, which is available nearly worldwide, has now been banned in France and Denmark. Its ingredients include, among other things: sucrose, glucose, sodium citrates, taurine, glucuronolactone, caffeine, niacin, vitamin B6, vitamin B12, flavouring and colours (caramel, riboflavin). Although mostly water, one can contains 27g of sugar (that's nine sugar lumps) and 80mg of caffeine (comparable to two cups of instant coffee).

Although this drink is marketed as an energy drink, it is hard to find one reason why any responsible sports person would drink it.

Fruit And Vegetable Juices

Raw fruit and vegetable juices do most of the excellent jobs that solid raw foods do, but in a way that places minimum strain on the digestive system. The concentrated vitamins, minerals, trace elements, enzymes, sugars and proteins they contain are absorbed into the bloodstream almost as soon as they reach the stomach and small intestine. Again it goes without saying, organic and biodynamic produce are best. Use a blender that doesn't overheat or it will render the juices nutritionless. An excellent choice of blender is a make called Oscar.

A freshly squeezed fruit juice two or three times a week, two hours either side of food, is delicious as well as nutritious. Two good combinations are: two oranges to one lemon; and one orange to a quarter grapefruit. (These mixtures counteract each other's acids.) There are obviously many more choices – just check your fruits against the food combining chart on www.lifesmart.co.uk to see if they are compatible digestively. Also take into account any allergies, candida, arthritis, migraine or any other severe pain in the skull and neck area. And check your skin, internal yeast content, gastric problems etc. as some fruits can irritate.

If you have problems with your skin, for example, avoid pineapple and berries as they are acidic and act as direct irritants to the skin, as well as aggravating cystitis and other urinary problems.

If you are constipated, avoid bananas as they are known to be binding to some people's systems. They are also a well-known allergen in people who have a sensitive digestive tract. However, they are an excellent energy source, aid the production of digestive enzymes and are high in several specific vitamins and minerals when eaten separately from main meals.

Do not eat too many apples – the pectin in apples is used as a gelling agent in foods and as a preservative in many jams, juices, dressings, packaged sauces and foods, which is just too much for any system to handle in such a consistently large amount. The pectin in apples can also irritate the bowels (constipation) and skin (spots, itching, rashes) and worsen cystitis and headaches.

Apples are great for fighting hunger pangs – but stick to the fruit itself (not every day), and aim to eat organic.

Individual or mixed vegetable and fruit juices can be delicious and nutritious – but make them yourself. Don't buy bottled juices as they tend to taste unpleasant and you don't know how long they've been sitting around for, building up yeast. Fresh juices mixed with carrot taste delicious. Don't forget your herbs – mixed with fruit juices they can add a real zing and are excellent for your system, or add your choice of herbs to juices in powder form.

Remedy Drinks

Fennel tea is good for aiding digestion; a teaspoon of organic cider vinegar in a glass of water, either hot or at room temperature, sipped half an hour after meals or throughout the day after a drinking or eating binge will help neutralize acids and make your system more alkaline – it also helps when any kind of toxic attack strikes such as stomach ache, headache or nausea. Celery leaves boiled in water and sipped for 20 minutes after meals help to reduce bloating.

Herbal Teas

Almost all herbal teas – and there is a vast range – are healthy. Check that the label says 'caffeine free'. Herbal teas have a number of healthy properties and are soothing while helping your body to digest food. Nettle tea is a great source of iron and is also a blood purifier and a kidney tonic. Fennel, peppermint and slippery elm teas all aid the digestive system and calm the stomach. Red raspberry leaf tea acts as a uterine toner and can relieve menstrual cramps. Instead of coffee try dandelion root coffee, a delicious, rich-tasting alternative – it's also a natural diuretic as well as being a liver tonic. It is even better if you buy all these teas in their natural loose form, giving your body extra help to clear out the toxins. The alternatives to regular coffee and tea are not only delicious but enormously beneficial to your health. Hot water and lemon juice is also very good for cleansing.

Go to www.lifesmart.co.uk for more advice on good foods to eat and an alternative shopping list of foodstuffs and ingredients.

Colds And Flu

Contrary to what you may believe, colds and flu are the body's way of getting rid of the toxins that build up from an overdose of yeast, sugar, antibiotics, lack of sleep or other negative behaviour that clogs up your system. This is your immune system letting you know that it's in good working order. If you are in good shape internally and externally, both mentally and physically, you will notice that no matter how many people are ill around you, it is unlikely that you will get ill. If, however, you are run down you will catch whatever is going.

If you have a cold or the flu, do not make the mistake of ingesting live yoghurt made from cow's milk (nor in this instance sheep's or goat's yoghurt), which will only block the mucus membranes further, exacerbating the whole process of cold- and flu-like symptoms. Instead, once you are through the worst of the illness, use acidophilus and bifidus capsules or powder and mix into soya yoghurt or simply take them on their own. Apart from this, ensure you rest and sleep and don't medicate yourself with drugs or supplements. It is healthy for the body to breakdown occasionally in this way. Ordinary or Chinese herbs and homeopathy may be effective. Remember you are likely to benefit from such a thorough clear out, and this is a fantastic opportunity to begin a healthy regime.

Losing Weight

If losing weight is your aim, there are a few rules you need to make with yourself in order to succeed and maintain your results.

1. Be realistic about the time it's going to take. Don't be fixated with the idea of losing weight quickly. Your body needs a decent amount of time to heal and adjust to a new eating programme, let alone lose weight. Your metabolism will have to sort itself out and your internal systems will have to learn how to function efficiently again.

2. Make a list of the excuses that you are likely to use which will hinder your long-term results, such as: not wanting to draw attention to yourself; stress; travelling; fatigue; depression; failing at work; anger; jealousy; boredom; dissatisfaction and apathy in any area of your life. Remember, every time you cheat, or stop and start, your body's ability to heal itself and to get into balance becomes weaker and weaker.

3 Organize your home and work environments so that you have a clear mind and a pleasant space to go back and forth to. This includes getting up to date on all administration and finances and any area that could cause you stress.

Put simply, it's up to you to keep to the rules – no one else has any control over your actions when it comes to caring for yourself. Nurture your ability to define and do what is necessary to attain all that you want. Always take notice of how you feel first and foremost, how you look second, and the scales last, or not at all.

The good news is that each person feels a huge weight has been lifted when bad habits are confronted. It's up to each individual to discover his or her problem and then to decide how to deal with it. And that includes the very sick. In fact, it's those suffering from cancer or multiple sclerosis, for example, who are often the least dramatic, sulky, self-righteous or indignant, and take full responsibility for changing their eating and drinking habits.

I know that losing weight and maintaining it, and overcoming problems such as obesity, anorexia or bulimia, or simply long-standing habits, are extremely hard. But when you consider how unwell you may have felt and for such a considerable time, isn't it worth expending your time and energy to achieve a balanced and healthy lifestyle?

• One in 10 primary school children is obese, double the figure of 20 years ago.

Action checklist

1. Decide the extent to which you are prepared to change your habits.
2. Look at how to make any new lifestyle work for you, not against you.
3. Be aware of which everyday emotions, events and excuses lead you to abuse yourself by eating and drinking badly.
4. Ask for people's help and understanding as you switch from bad habits to good, especially your partner's. And certainly never use people or their negative attitudes as a reason not to be able to do what you want where healthy nutrition is concerned.
5. Make a plan to see you through the time it will take you to achieve your goal.

Before you do anything, sit down with a piece of paper and list what you can remember about the food you ate between the ages of five and 20 and from 20 to now. In particular note any tinned foods, semolina and other rice puddings, supermarket cereals, pasta, fried breakfasts, chips, bread, red meat, salads and vegetables covered in salad cream or butter, salt on food, cakes and chocolate, rich foreign food, processed meats, sugar, additives, preservatives, vinegar, dairy produce, pastry, fish fingers and frozen fish.

You may become aware that while you were growing up, most of your food was either processed, high in fats, salt and sugar or generally low in nutritional value. This is why in the adult years people's immune systems are so often dysfunctional.

Whatever regime you may be following, you must recognize three priorities:

1. That you stick to all the rules on hydration and liquids.
2. That your alkaline content remains between 70 and 80 per cent of your food intake each meal.

3. That for those of you who struggle with digestion or are below par in any way, food combining during the working week can help ease digestion. This is also a great way to limit over eating.

Also, get to know the glycaemic index (see page 88) – it helps to keep your cravings, metabolic rate and thyroid in control.

Conclusion

The purpose of bothering to eat healthily has to encompass all the different aspects of your life: your love life, career, emotional well-being, relaxation, self-confidence, children, friends and so on. If you honed in on just one trigger point that could keep you in line, you may just change the personal pattern of a lifetime. At the end of the day, the best way of eating is to have a cross-section of all the foods that are good for you. The key to nutrition is thinking carefully about what you eat, planning a day's meals so that all the nutrients you require are included, changing the habits of a lifetime and genuinely wanting to make changes to the way you look, feel, act and view things.

Good nutrition is not always easy ... to begin with. Once you get the ball rolling it becomes easier and easier, and much more fun! And when the compliments start pouring in, when your skin, hair, teeth and nails become stronger and healthier, and when your health problems start fading away, there'll be no stopping you. So good luck, grab your shopping list and get started.

Physical Pursuits

THE FITNESS INDUSTRY HAS had as many fads as the diet industry. Each comes with a set of promises that will right every wrong, and there has been much mud slinging between and even within the different exercise regimes and philosophies. Contraindications and varying teaching methods have been the main causes for this rivalry.

However, recently these prejudices and barriers have largely disappeared. Of the 26 years that I have been teaching, 10 have been in a gym environment. In the early days I was frowned upon for mixing Pilates, ballet bar, yoga, core and isolation techniques with cardiovascular and resistance training, but thankfully this has now changed. It is gratifying to see some of the younger trainers and old die-hards of the industry representing a new breed of trainers who are drawing on a cross-section of influences both within and outside of the gym culture. The truth is that every 'body' needs a variety of skills, exercises and pace in order to service their own physical needs and goals. So, even though the newspapers in recent times have criticized gyms for being one-dimensional and a poor substitute for exercising outdoors, you can derive an enormous amount from the mix that is available in gyms today.

Whatever your chosen exercise, it is crucial for you to have the confidence and understanding to execute any form of physical exercise correctly. Busy mothers who need crèche facilities, business people who travel a lot, sports-specific skills, remedial exercises, technique and weather constraints in many countries make the modern-day gym essential to the continuity of our health and fitness.

So What's Putting Us Off?

Laziness and boredom are obvious factors in the reluctance to exercise. However, the real cause often stems from school days, when having been thrown into competitive games that were skills-orientated, many children felt intimidated. As a result a number of people are put off physical activity at a very young age. I would say that the vast majority of personal training clients and latecomers to exercising fall into this category.

Breathing, posture, preliminary coordination and isolation skills (working different muscles independently of others) as well as learning about the different muscle groups weren't (and still aren't) a part of the school sports curriculum.

In addition, we're frightened of making fools of ourselves and failing. The images in all the magazines and books are very slick and a world away from how a lot of people see themselves. I hear stories of people going for their first assessment at a gym and having inexperienced personnel foisted on them, or tales of people being crushingly bored. As a result they give up the idea of using a gym for exercising.

Many personal training books, trainers and fitness instructors concentrate on putting pressure on people to be constantly motivated and goal driven. I know that it is done with the best of intentions, but with the general exhaustion, stress levels and physical dysfunction present today, the 'burn mentality' on its own is no longer appropriate. I believe it's much more beneficial for you to naturally aspire to improving your exercise capabilities without feeling constantly forced.

Moving Forward

As an ex-dancer and sufferer of a chronic back condition that left me 80 per cent immobile for three years, I truly empathize with anyone who hates the idea of having to do what seems like contrived exercise. However, had I not been shamed into doing something about my own predicament I would never have moved on.

Being able to move without restriction is a luxury that does not belong to everyone. It still baffles me that, with life expectancy longer than it has ever been before, inactivity in the Western world has not only escalated, but is also breeding old bodies before their time. We still seem to accept that old age equals physical decline and general immobility. Yet, if you look at the small percentage of 60- to 90-year-olds who incorporate flexibility, posture, strength work and walking into their daily lives, they are vital and alert with excellent posture and certainly do not look anywhere near their age.

Arsenal Football Club

We idolize famous footballers, sporting heroes, models and celebrities, not just for their looks, but for their physical prowess. Yet when you go to a football or tennis match the crowd is full of people who clearly don't emulate their heroes' penchant for physical pursuits. In fact the consumption of alcohol, fast food and cigarettes seems worse than ever at these types of event. Perhaps we can take inspiration from the new regimes being introduced by club managers such as Arsenal's Arsene Wenger.

Not many people know about the specific regimes that the players adhere to in order to be spectacular throughout the match period. Stamina, fitness levels, flexibility and stretching allow a player of any sport to have an edge on their opponent due to their extra speed, agility, ability to coordinate and potential for their muscles to repair, both in terms of injury and from normal wear and tear.

In the old days training was all about track and stamina with laps, star jumps and press-ups. But today a player's training has become far more scientific and holistic.

For example, since Wenger came to England and became the manager of the Arsenal Football club he has introduced a whole new approach to the way players are trained. At the Arsenal training facility at London Colney the players are assessed individually. Each player's nutrition and exercise is tailored to their specific needs and requirements. Their psychological needs are also catered for with stress-management techniques and ongoing support. When any injuries occur a wide range of techniques is available not only to repair the injury as quickly as possible but also to limit any long-term damage.

This 'whole person' approach obviously works as can be seen not only from the results being achieved by the club but also by listening to the individual players who have nothing but praise for Wenger and the Arsenal staff for the physical and mental well-being they have attained.

Exercise And Instructions

In this chapter I am going to concentrate on some dos and don'ts and correct technique that will be beneficial to both beginners and seasoned exercisers. You will see examples of men and women ranging in age from 16 to 70. Apart from my mother, I have picked a mixture of people, most of whom I have not worked with before, to show teaching points and problems that you may relate to. **Their case histories and all the exercises and accompanying instructions are on www.lifesmart.co.uk so you can incorporate them when you are working out.**

Types Of Exercisers

Often people who lack muscle memory and confidence, as a result of never liking (let alone participating in) physical activities, suffer one of two exercise-related malaises. The first is dyspraxia, which is the physical equivalent of dyslexia. As a result fitness, stamina and strength as goals have to be relegated to secondary importance in order to develop mobility, isolation and body-eye coordination skills first. All other skills and physical pursuits fall into place far more easily as a result.

Other people may have difficulty focusing on the whole physical aspect of what they are doing and can be quite lazy. The trainer has to work harder, constantly pushing the person to keep them motivated. It's always important to remember that exercise is 75 per cent intention and mental orientation and 25 per cent physical output. Your attention to detail as to how you perform an exercise and what you get out of it is of prime importance.

Using a wobble board is a great way to get people focused on their bodies. Many people remark that it is the nearest they have felt to being grounded and find it strangely relaxing. The wobble board concentrates on building core and joint stability, posture and balance. Touch training, which is where the trainer uses his hand and also yours to feel what muscles you are working or to provide resistance instead of a weight or a machine, is also beneficial in this instance.

• 63 per cent of men and 75 per cent of women fail to meet the current UK government recommendations of doing at least 30 minutes of moderate intensity activity five or more days a week.

Those who are self-motivated do a very good job of putting in the time and the effort but often, apart from building cardiovascular endurance and increased strength, technique can be hugely lacking. They also often don't tackle posture, stretching, core stability or isolation. For those of you who fall into this category (and it is a majority), spend a couple of weeks watching the personal trainers in your gym to determine the ones who are skills-specific and who work on these areas, then book a couple of sessions with them. Developing the skills to be visually cognizant and to be able to feel when your positions and movements are incorrect are crucial to the whole feel and outcome of any physical activity. You will get immense input that will add a whole new dimension and, of course, results to your workouts.

Variety

Variety is the spice of life! Your body is no different from your brain, it needs a certain amount of continuity, but it is also very quick to adjust to the strains of a new regime.

For cardiovascular exercise, make sure you don't end up using one machine for the same amount of time each day until you plateau. You may find you damage your muscles or joints in the process and you will dilute your chances of attaining the goals you may have set for yourself.

The two main types of cardiovascular exercise are either weight-bearing or non-weight-bearing. Weight-bearing is where your feet and legs support your body weight, and is great for strengthening your bones. Examples include walking, running, stair master, skipping and cross trainer. Non-weight-bearing is where your torso is supported, tending to make life easier for your back, knees or other joints. These exercises include cycling, rowing and swimming.

Doing a mixture of these activities, at different points of your workout, coupled with varying the programmes, speed and time, will ensure that your body always rises to the challenge. Some days it is equally appropriate to skip cardiovascular exercises altogether and just perform mat and floor work, concentrating on flexibility, toning, stomach, back and strength work.

Preparing the muscles for strenuous exercise by gradually warming up and cooling down for five to 10 minutes will protect the heart and decrease the chance of muscle strains and injuries as well as preventing soreness, cramping, dizziness and lightheadedness.

If you are a yoga or Pilates aficionado you will know that warming up does not involve any cardiovascular activity, and stretching and breathing is used in its place. This is another way of creating variety if you are predominantly a gym goer who focuses on cardiovascular exercise. Start your sessions with stretches and breathing exercises, especially if your energy levels and immune system are flagging, or for women who are about to start their monthly cycle. This is also helpful for men who go into their workouts completely knotted up and tense from the day. Every male client I have taught over the last 25 years has vastly

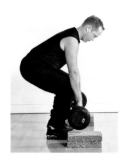

Like most men, Michael focuses solely on cardio and upper body weight training. Here he is doing a dumbbell bar squat concentrating on keeping his vertebrae, arms, knees and feet in correct alignment. For specific teaching points and other lower body exercises go to www.lifesmart.co.uk.

benefited from this. You can start off by stretching on the bar, followed by mat work or an upper body workout and if, during the course of the session, you feel like incorporating or finishing off with cardiovascular exercise you can. You will find that your capacity for other exercise is greater, just through opening up the body, stretching the muscle fibres throughout and activating the lymph, and because you have varied your habits.

Traditionally, women have gone for the gentler, more stretching types of exercise such as yoga and Pilates, while men have concentrated on weight training and cardiovascular workouts. Today that is rapidly changing. Women have made great strides in weight-bearing and cardiovascular exercise, but we still have a long way to go in getting the numbers up in women of all ages. Men have made progress by including more variety but they still need to concentrate on balancing out their upper body work with lower body weight training and stretches. Everybody can derive huge benefit from incorporating core stability and balance work, martial arts, remedial bar work and isolation training, amongst others, into their regimes.

When it comes to strength training it's equally important to use a mixture of resistance machines, free weights, cable machine and your own body resistance. During any weight-training routine go for a lesser weight and concentrate on increasing the repetitions on days when you are feeling weak or tired. At other times progressively increase the amount of weight lifted as this will cause the body to adapt to the increase in demand by adding lean muscle tissue.

The secret is to achieve a balance between being consistent in order to improve while keeping your body guessing at what's coming next. Your muscles don't have eyes, so they can only interpret movement. For example, by switching from a linear walking motion to a rotary movement while cycling, you are forcing your body to adapt. This will not only bring about results but it will also enhance your sessions by preventing boredom and the overuse of the same muscles and joints. Plus you are training your brain to be more adaptable.

Preparing Yourself

If you really want to give yourself a head start, why not have a comprehensive medical? It's a good way of focusing on the overall picture.

Whether you are a seasoned exerciser or not, it is a good idea to have one or two cranial-osteopathic sessions in order to check that everything is as it should be, and to better understand your body – particularly those areas that are most tense. Posture isn't just the way that you stand; it's also the way that your limbs hang from your body so each has a posture and an alignment of its own. All this can be pointed out to you by a good osteopath and can help you develop essential know-how that is specific to your structure.

It is also useful to check your diet with a professional. If you are having any difficulties with your digestive system, headaches or energy levels, the personalized information you receive can usually determine the degree of impact-based aerobic training you are or aren't able to manage within your first three months. If, for example, your colon is quite congested and you get regular indigestion, stomach cramps and irritable bowel you may be better off doing non-impact aerobics at first where you are not landing in such a way as to aggravate the problem area. Once your body has acclimatized you should have no problem in including more impact-based work.

If possible, when starting out on a new exercise regime I would highly recommend four personal training sessions with an experienced all-round personal trainer over the course of a month. Doing this will make the world of difference to your desired outcome. Learning correct techniques will establish correct habits, eliminate bad ones, and can be used in any exercise environment.

As soon as you create heat within the muscle through sweating and physical exertion you activate two systems. One is your emotional memory and the other is your elimination system. It's good to be aware of this before you start out, so that if you feel anxious, irritated, weepy or slightly nauseous you will know not to be worried or take it too seriously. All you have to do is breathe through it and take it slowly, stopping if you need to. It doesn't often occur but it's good to be prepared. Breathing alone can help the system expel all sorts of emotional and physical debris.

Clothing should always be made of natural fibres. Nylon is a popular material but does not allow your skin to breathe — you will know yourself as the odour that comes from nylon is far greater than from cotton, for example. Clothing should not be restrictive or make you feel self-conscious; at the same time you want to wear something where you can see what the general outline of your body is doing. Always make sure you are warm enough at first with layers you can peel off.

When you begin to exercise, as with losing weight, you can often hit against a personal brick wall. You may feel that you are getting nowhere, but progress is taking place as the muscles in your body are starting to realign and correct themselves. When you least expect it you will be able to perform certain exercises that you found particularly hard, or make a leap of improvement in other areas.

Conversely, when the body changes we are quick to forget the progress that has been made. The body doesn't just expand continuously, it expands and contracts and goes up and down in terms of energy levels, stamina and ability.

(Left) Beginner's position of static hamstring stretch. (Centre) Once the muscle is fully warmed up, a combination of bending and straightening the knee, with hands strategically placed to ease the back of your legs out, results in increased flexibility. (Below) An advanced position. Extending both legs a little bit further as the muscles expand their range of flexibility.

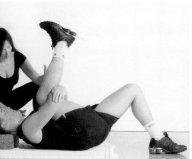
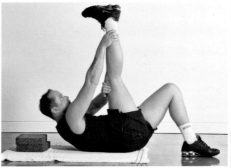
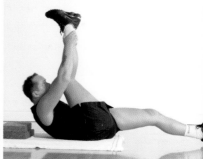

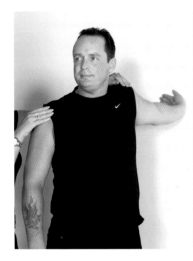
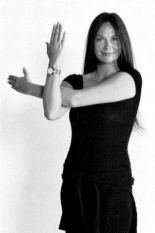
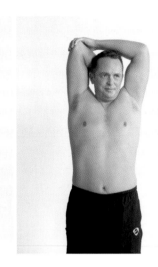

A selection of upper body stretches. These should be done before, in between, and after weight training different areas of the upper body. (Above) Stretching the pectoral and biceps (across the chest and along front of arm). (Centre) Stretching the deltoids (shoulders). (Above right) Stretching the triceps (back of arm).

Comparing Your Performance

When it comes to exercising, some people knowingly or otherwise judge themselves against others. Men do it with weights, thinking that the heavier the better and that bulk and size are priority. They don't take into account their body frames or the capacity of the body part they are working, often stressing the muscle fibres which can eventually lead to repetitive strain injuries.

Women often compare themselves to other women in terms of their flexibility. If they see somebody who can get their head on their knees, while they are struggling, they immediately think there's no point even trying as they are never going to be able to achieve that. However, stretching is designed to relax the tendons and muscles, reduce stress to the joints, dissipate lactic acid, increase blood flow to repair muscle fibres and to promote the flow of oxygen and blood throughout the body. So stretching effectively doesn't rely on performance, it just relies on you doing it.

Overriding Injury And Illness

Very often those who exercise regularly will override injury, illness and exhaustion. This is very common and borders on the obsessive. Of course, instead of the body being the beneficiary as the participant thinks, it is in fact the antithesis, resulting in the body becoming less able to recover and repair itself. Similar to crash dieting, there is only so much your body is able to undertake and, like any system, if you continuously override it, there will come a point when it will not be able to sustain such output.

Pushing your body by exercising when you feel a cold or sore throat coming on is counter-productive. The immune system is compromised as all it wants to do is fight the infection. All you are achieving by continuing to exercise is circulating the infection or virus throughout your lymphatic system, making recovery much harder and courting ongoing minor illnesses and a weakened immune system.

My advice is that you go to bed, drink plenty of water and let your system recuperate. As you begin to recover do only very gentle stretching and mat work and slowly ease back into your routine. Where injuries are concerned, if you don't allow for a full recovery, no matter how small the injury, you run the risk of permanent damage.

Recovery in exercise is very important. The changes in the muscles that you are trying to acquire take place during rest time, and because so many regimes are goal-orientated they all have different recommendations for how often, how long and at what capacity you should be training. Feeling the fruits of your endeavours is a good sign, but sustaining continual lactic acid build up, soreness and shaking is not. Your rest, food and water intake must be complementary to your output, and if you miss a week you will benefit if nothing else from the change in routine.

Backs And Structural Injuries

Warming up using cardiovascular activity really doesn't apply when it comes to structural problems. Once you have had a proper diagnosis as to what is wrong, it is crucial to understand how the problem area is affected by different types of activities and movements and how the rest of the body is affected by the problem area.

A sensible place to start is to follow specially prescribed corrective exercises that follow the spider's web of the whole body, often starting with static stretching to release and expand tight muscle fibres followed by tiny contractive movements for strengthening specific muscles.

If you have a weak or immobile back or suffer from everyday discomfort, you need to check that your bed or your seating at work and in the car are not partly causing or aggravating the problem. In order for backs to be worked comprehensively you have to use correct posture, breathing, mobility, isolation and core stability in order to eradicate any discrepancies.

Email info@londonspineclinic.com for details on The London Spine Clinic who specialize in all structural problems.

(Below left) A beginner's glut stretch. (Centre) The beginner's way of stretching the outer sections and front of the quad. (Below) Everyone who does yoga knows the reclining hero position. Most people find this particularly hard, and it can result in compromising the knee joints and base of spine. Carole shows Pearl what steps to take to reach full hero position safely.

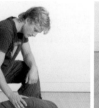
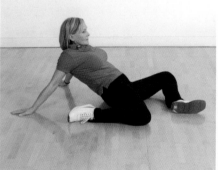
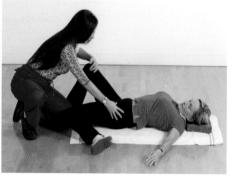

Exercise, Alcohol And Smoking

Many people believe that if they exercise hard enough it will minimize the damage that alcohol and smoking does to the body. This of course is not the case. It's no coincidence that some of the most ferocious workouts are done by people who ingest these substances.

Endorphins are a hormone that share a similar biochemical reaction to drugs and alcohol. That is why recovering addicts, heavy drinkers and regular smokers have to be extremely careful in their choice and quantity of cardiovascular output and overdoing any form of exercise. While it is crucial that they take some exercise it shouldn't be anything that will loop them back into using their chosen substance.

A day hardly goes by in the gym when I don't see some of the regulars lighting up a cigarette, eating food crammed with sugar (like chocolate), or drinking energy drinks, colas or coffee, even before they get through the front doors. The truth is that they are putting an incredible strain on their heart and lungs in particular, and also their liver and nervous system. Of course it's better than doing nothing and they are unlikely to be confronted by any teacher or trainer. But that doesn't mean to say that they can get away with it in the long run. Despite what you believe, internal damage, ageing and a weak immune system will not be deterred through exercise alone…

Fat Loss Versus Weight Reduction

As much as I don't want to make fat and weight the most important issue of the day, they can't be ignored. Too many people listen to the myths and don't fully understand the facts about their body shape and weight.

It's easy to get confused between weight loss and fat loss; however, they are not the same. Excess fat tissue is what makes you look flabby and can be tackled by using exercise to burn the fat. Weight loss from sensible eating, on the other hand, will lose you fat in terms of poundage, but this does not deal with the loose fatty tissue that is often left as a residue after losing a substantial amount of weight.

In order to lose body fat tissue, apart from any recommended changes to your diet, you have to use a mixture of aerobic activity and weight-bearing exercise. See www.lifesmart.co.uk for more information.

Body Fat Distribution

Your body shape determines the distribution of your body fat. Being overweight or having too much excess body fat is bad for your health, but total body fat is not the only health risk. Body fat distribution is also significant.

If, according to the Body Mass Index, you are overweight but your weight is evenly distributed over your body or concentrated below the waist then your health risks are greatly reduced. On the other hand, research has shown that excess weight concentrated around the abdomen is a much higher health risk than excess weight located below the waist on the hips, bottom or thighs.

• Between 1980 and 2002, the number of obese men in the UK rose from 6 per cent to 22 per cent. For women, the figure increased from 8 per cent to 23 per cent.

Body Types

Our body types are genetically determined from birth and actually have more to do with bone structure and the body's frame than the muscle tissue itself. Although we cannot alter our body type, everyone has the physical potential to develop a great shape through correct diet and exercise. It's simply the case that each body type responds differently to both training and nutrition.

There are three basic categories of body type: ectomorph, endomorph and mesomorph. Most people display a mixture of body types such as ecto-mesomorphs or endo-mesomorphs, but one type is usually dominant.

Ectomorphs are characterized by a thin, linear appearance and their physique is fragile and delicate. They often possess a narrow waist, hips and shoulders and a low body fat percentage. Their downfall is the lack of shape due to low muscle weight. The ectomorph is not naturally powerful and will have to work hard for every ounce of muscle and strength. Ectomorphs are encouraged to add extra calories (favouring carbohydrates) while consuming ample amounts of protein. When using weights, intensely productive sets are required to promote muscle growth.

Endomorphs are characterized by big bones, a high waist and usually a high degree of body fat around the midsection and thighs. They tend to have more internal fat deposits lining the organs, making it harder to lose weight, which they find a constant struggle. They need to develop a higher degree of motivation to produce the drive required to lose weight by using correct nutrition and exercise that will burn fat effectively. Endomorphs need to cut dietary fat down to a minimum and eat lean protein. Small portions and frequent meals will help boost the metabolism. Plenty of cardiovascular exercise is required to keep the weight down and weight training should be moderate with sets of several repetitions.

Mesomorphs tend to have the best attributes of both the ectomorphs and the endomorphs and are characterized by broad shoulders, well-defined muscles, large bones, a relatively narrow low waist and a fast metabolism due to the amount of lean muscle. Mesomorphs do need to follow a healthy diet and exercise programme, but they should be able to maintain their physiques by following general guidelines.

Spot Reducing

As you can see, your gender and genetic make-up will determine where your body lays down fat. In addition, it determines from where the body chooses to draw fat for fuel. Spot reducing through exercise alone is pointless because many of us try to reduce areas that are just a natural part of our physical package. Most men, for example, store fat around their middle, which leads to the so-called 'love handles' or 'spare tyre'. Most women store fat on their hips and thighs.

The number of fat cells that each person has is constant throughout their life. Fat cells don't break down – the cells simply deflate as the fat is squeezed out;

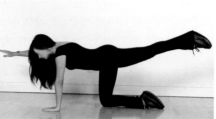
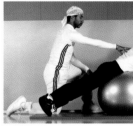

A mixture of remedial back and core stability exercises.

as weight is gained the cells plump up again. Because the skin is elastic, as you put on weight the skin is stretched. If you lose weight rapidly then the skin will collapse and sag. It is therefore imperative to lose weight gradually by drinking lots of water, eating lots of fibre and cutting back on sugar and refined foods. Along with weight training and aerobic activity, which will raise your metabolic rate, you will become a more efficient fat-burning machine and will hopefully never require a surgical skin tuck!

Raising Your Metabolic Rate

Given that we are stuck with our genes, age and gender, there are some parts of the metabolic equation that we are also stuck with! We can, however, boost our metabolism – the speed at which calories are burned – and one of the best ways to do this is to replace the fat we're carrying around with lean tissue in both the big and small muscles. Muscle at rest requires fuel so the more muscle, the more fuel needed – and the more calories you burn. So, even when you are enjoying some time off from the gym your hard work is still paying off. Replacing fat with muscle requires a combination of aerobic activity, muscle-building weight workouts and changes to your diet.

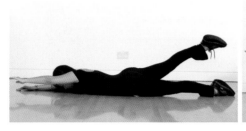

Michael Button when he was 17 stone. He is now 13 stone and demonstrates a number of the exercises in this chapter.

CASE STUDY – MICHAEL BUTTON

Four years ago Michael was fairly stable at 12 ½ stone, but after giving up smoking he rocketed to 17 stone. He began to notice how the extra weight he was carrying made him tired from walking just a few hundred yards. At night his feet ached, he looked and felt like Homer Simpson and his friends and work colleagues were constantly making fun of him.

Michael realized that he needed to do something about the situation, so he joined a gym where he received an initial consultation with a trainer. Together they ran through his goals, how they wanted to achieve them and in what timescale, and Michael began a routine that enabled him to lose the first stone.

At 15 stone Michael hit a wall; he couldn't seem to shift any more weight. After speaking to the gym staff he changed his routine and again began to lose weight. His body had simply adapted to his routine and needed to be challenged further. He then lost a further two stone and reached his goal of 13 stone.

Michael has now switched his focus from cardiovascular work to building up lean muscle mass and stretching, but still keeps cardiovascular exercises in his routine. He admits that his present fitness involved a lot of hard work but that the results have affected every facet of his life. He sees the difference in the way people interact with him and he feels happier and more positive than he ever has before.

The Cardiovascular System

The cardiovascular system includes the heart, blood vessels and respiratory system, and is responsible for carrying oxygen from the air to the bloodstream and for expelling the waste product of carbon dioxide. By performing exercise the body's overall cardiovascular endurance and efficiency will improve. The lungs will begin to process more air with less effort, the heart to pump more blood with fewer beats, and there will be an increase of blood to the muscles.

The body uses two different systems to supply energy to the muscles — aerobic and anaerobic, both of which are needed for the development of physical fitness.

The term 'aerobic' means with air or oxygen. Oxygen is essential for muscles to function correctly, allowing them to extract all the energy they require from blood sugar. Aerobic exercise comprises any activity using large muscle groups rhythmically and sustainably for an extended period of time. It elevates the heart rate and breathing, but note that while doing aerobic exercise you should be able to maintain a short conversation without gasping for air.

Anaerobic on the other hand means without air or oxygen. The workouts are of a higher intensity and for a shorter duration due to the lack of oxygen and the build-up of lactic acid which contributes to muscle fatigue. This type of exercise helps to increase muscle strength and is relied on for quick, short bursts of speed. However, it requires a recovery period for the lactic acid to be burned up by the body and for the muscles to use oxygen for replenishing energy.

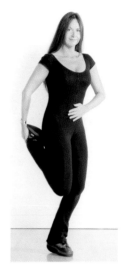

Two different quad stretches emphasizing correct position of spine and pelvis, and alignment of knees in Carole's example (above), and right angle of front leg in Michael's (below).

Aerobic Exercise And The Fat-burning Myth

While doing aerobic exercise the body will always use up a combination of fat and carbohydrate. The question is what will burn more, a low-, medium- or high-intensity workout? It doesn't matter if you're burning a little extra fat or a little extra carbohydrate. The bottom line is how many overall calories are burned. To lose weight you need to burn more calories than your body consumes and utilizes every day.

It is also interesting to see how low-, medium- and high-intensity workouts burn fat or carbohydrates. You actually initially burn more fat during a low-intensity workout. However, in the same time period with a high-intensity workout you will burn more total calories and therefore more fat overall as shown in the following table:

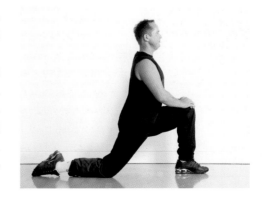

30 MINUTES ACTIVITY	CALORIES BURNED	FAT PERCENTAGE	CALORIES FROM FAT
Reading a Newspaper	40	60 %	24
Walking	100	65 %	65
Jogging	350	40 %	100

So why choose a low-intensity workout over a high-intensity one? Because it takes time for a beginner to build up the physical ability to work at this pace, to avoid exhaustion, and to minimize the increased risk of injury any high-intensity activity involves.

I recommend a mixture of low-, medium- and high-intensity exercises, bearing in mind all the different factors such as how much time you have, your goals, how you feel and so on. Just remember that moderate intensity increases your basal metabolic rate (BMR) more than lower intensity so you are consistently burning more calories.

All the information you need regarding basal metabolic rate (BMR); resting heart rate (RHR); blood pressure; body mass index (BMI); target heart rate zone (THR); Borg rating of perceived exertion exercise; exercise for older people and during pregnancy can be found at www.lifesmart.co.uk.

CASE STUDY – LESLIE HILL

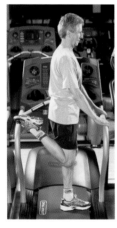

Leslie Hill is 67 years old and over the last 20 years has held posts such as the Chairman of ITV, Chairman of Central Television and most recently as the Managing Director of EMI Music Europe. Long hours and high stress involved in his career, along with a lack of exercise led to him becoming overweight. By the time he retired 10 years ago he had joined nearly half the adult population in the UK who suffer from lower back pain.

Visiting a physiotherapist he was told to stop his sporadic outside running and to replace it with a gym treadmill. So began Leslie's love affair with the gym and he now works out most weekdays and perfects his techniques with a personal trainer twice a week. Not only has he lost the excess weight but he feels more invigorated and looks better than he did at half his age. Leslie stresses the importance of exercising, not only for keeping trim and fit but also for keeping mentally alert.

Leslie using the walking machine to support and advance this quadricep stretch.

As you can see, it's not just young people who need to exercise; there are also major benefits for the older generation. It is safe to start exercising at an advanced age as long as it is done correctly and built up slowly. Benefits include the lowering of blood pressure and blood sugar, improved cholesterol levels and the slowing down of the onset or development of osteoporosis.

As you get older you lose 20 to 40 per cent of your muscle tissue. Again this is something that can be remedied by doing strength and resistance training. Increased muscle strength can protect vulnerable joints and improve flexibility, coordination and balance. With a lack of regular exercise the human body's ability to function will decline, making daily activities extremely difficult and often resulting in the need of carers to perform even simple tasks.

At www.lifesmart.co.uk you can find information about all the exercises and equipment in this section.

Cardiovascular Equipment

There really is no 'best' cardiovascular activity. I would recommend a balanced mixture, taking any injuries into account, in order to maximize results.

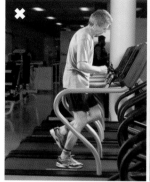
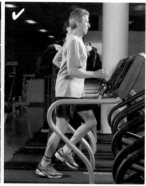

Treadmill

How you walk is of prime importance. Far too many walkers have bad posture: rounded shoulders, collapsed diaphragms, landing heavily on their feet with arms swinging loosely.

(Above left) Incorrect posture and technique for walking and running. (Above) Correct posture and technique for walking and running.

Leslie (above) demonstrates both incorrect and correct techniques. Using correct posture described on page 149, with arms bent at a right angle, move back and forth in rhythm with your legs. Use wide strides concentrating on leading with your pelvis, which will engage your adductor muscles (inner thighs). Keep your feet facing forward (many people have a tendency to turn their feet out).

Low-impact Exercises

For walkers and runners alike, injuries are common from the constant pounding of joints on asphalt and concrete. Good treadmills offer surfaces that absorb impact and reduce pressure, so injuries are less common and stress on critical joints is reduced. Achilles tendons, knee joints, back muscles, ankles and thighs take less of a pounding, which guarantees that you'll continue to walk or run into your old age. For an extra challenge wear MBT trainers while exercising.

For recommendations of sportswear see www.lifesmart.co.uk.

(Below left) Incorrect posture and technique on the cross trainer. (Below) Correct posture and technique on the cross trainer.

Cross Trainer

Cross or elliptical trainers combine the natural stride of walking on a treadmill and the motion of a stair climber. On an elliptical trainer, you stand comfortably in an upright position while holding on to the machine's handrails and striding in either a forward or reverse motion (see right for correct and incorrect positions).

What makes this machine unique is the ability to offer a weight-bearing workout that puts minimal stress on the joints. Your feet never leave the pedals of an elliptical trainer,

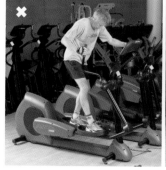
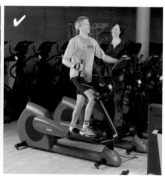

thereby eliminating any impact. Whether you go forward or in reverse, and regardless of the level of resistance or participant's age, the risk of injury is reduced from overusing any one muscle group, at the same time as providing a full upper and lower body workout.

Cross trainers appeal to a population that is increasingly overweight and looking for an optimum workout for burning fat and calories, without risking injury or discomfort.

Stationary Bike

This is another easy piece of equipment to start out on without the impact on joints of a treadmill. Here are a few things to keep in mind when working out:

Adjust the seat to your body. When you sit on the cycle's seat with your foot on the pedal in its lowest position, there should be only a slight bend in your knee, approximately 25–35 degrees.

Watch your form. Pay close attention to your upper body and don't slouch over the handlebars. Keep your torso lifted, your shoulders relaxed and your head looking straight ahead. If you're really getting into your ride and want to vary the intensity, crank up the resistance *and* pedal while standing out of your seat. It adds variety and helps prevent a sore bottom. The reclining bike is excellent for supporting a perfect posture and focuses solely on your lower body. Whichever bike you choose, ideally keep the rpm's at a minimum of 70 and an average of between 80 and 90. As this becomes comfortable you can increase the resistance, time and distance…

Rowing Machine

Many people think this machine is only good for the upper body, but that's not true. Rowing targets both the upper and lower body muscles, with the benefit of cultivating correct upper body posture, although people are not being taught correctly, or corrected when they use the machine. Flicking wrists, using momentum by throwing the torso back and forward, flaccid grip and not completing the movement at either end are just some of the strange habits that I've seen.

To row with the correct technique, sit down and slide your bottom back so that your back is upright, with your chest slightly leaning forward. Grab the handle at either end in an overhand grip and slide the seat forward until your legs are bent at a little more than 90 degrees and your arms are straight out in front of you. Now, push with your legs and when they're almost straight, pull the handle to just below your chest level. Keep your elbows tucked close to your side. Your back should be upright with little movement throughout the exercise other than to stretch as fully as possible on the forward part of the movement. To release, straighten your arms, then bend your knees after the handle clears them and slowly glide forward to the starting position. You will soon get into a rhythm. Make sure each movement is strong and full and once you are confident you can alter your grip and speed accordingly.

Rowing is one of the most complete cardiovascular exercises around. A proper rowing routine will tone all of your major muscle groups in your legs, back and arms. It will also help increase your V02 max and increase your heartbeat. It is physically demanding, so you should start off slowly and gradually increase the resistance and duration of the sessions.

Rowing is very easy on the joints as, unlike running, it doesn't require any heavy pounding movements. It's important, however, to stretch your lower back before every session because of the movement's nature, which can be challenging to an inflexible or problematic lower spine. For the many people with disc problems, rowing is often not suitable as it can severely irritate your back and cause extra damage. Check with your physiotherapist or osteopath before you use a rowing machine.

Stairmaster

People with bad backs have to take particular care with this machine, and if in doubt skip this until your back is stronger. The trick is to stand as upright as possible, with your shoulders relaxed, your ribs lifted, your chest open and your arms straight with a small break at the elbow. Using the whole foot, move your weight alternately, concentrating on full, long, slow strides at first, and then try shortening the movements which will add speed. Alternate between the different paces. Breathing is particularly important. Try not to hold your breath or lean on the machine and slow down your breathing all the time. Start on a low level for a minimum of three minutes, then build both time and levels slowly.

Momentum Training

This can be seen in all areas of exercise and is the least productive, most dangerous way of working the body. Momentum training is often used to force the body to perform over and above its capability. This is cheating: in order to lift, push or pull a heavier weight, instead of having the discipline to execute the lift (or the stretch) through the targeted muscle group, other parts of the body

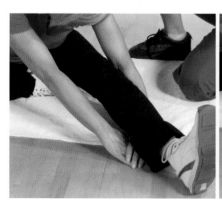 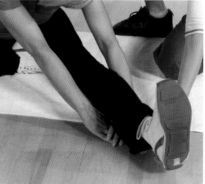

Pearl is practising a hamstring and spinal erector stretch but in such a way that she is contracting and strengthening the quadriceps and knee joints at the same time.

are used to compensate by employing a swinging motion. By doing this you are not developing the primary area adequately, and are also at risk of incurring injury and overdevelopment of the supporting muscle groups.

In stretching exercises, this is known as a ballistic movement, and can result in muscle strains or tears. The bouncing or flinging characteristic of this type of stretching motion actually elicits a reflexive contraction. The only time this is appropriate is if it is sports specific, such as for martial arts or ballet. I still think that it is better to have the patience to allow the muscle to reach the point of tension, and then you can allow the body to relax into the stretch either with slow, static stretching or a mixture of slow gentle pulses and rocking. Try doing this when following the exercises on page 147, alternating with a side-to-side rocking movement which has a massaging effect on the muscles, making sure you are breathing correctly throughout. Always hold a static stretch for at least 30 seconds. It's especially beneficial to repeat stretches, making sure you alternate between one side then the other.

When stretching your hamstrings, if you put one hand on top of the other then place them under your calf, the arms can be used as natural levers while bending and extending the knee alternately. After the first 20 seconds, gently pulse and rock from side to side to help ease out the muscles. Sitting on a yoga block can help those with stiff lower backs, yet add challenge to those who are very flexible.

Breathing And Posture

It goes without saying that general fitness is very important. However, learning to breathe and stand correctly is fundamental to all exercise, and even the most advanced exerciser may need to make substantial improvements. When you breathe fully without causing tension and stiffness to the upper body, the quality you add to any regime is dramatic. Oxygen levels, lymph and blood flow as well as stamina are increased considerably. In order to reach full capacity your thorax and diaphragm need to be fully extended and open.

Anyone suffering from indigestion or a headache at the start of exercising can, using a combination of correct posture, breathing, stretch and certain upper body weight-bearing exercises, eliminate these problems by the end of a session.

Breathing

Many people have problems when learning how to breathe correctly or perform any exercise, for that matter. The reason for this is that learning is mainly encouraged as an intellectual process. But with exercise, the emphasis should be on your ability to *feel* what you are doing and then to visually recognize whether you are performing the movements correctly or not.

There are many different philosophies that teach breathing, for example the Alexander Technique, yoga and Pilates. The trouble is that if you are not participating in any of these it is unlikely that you will be taught the benefits and the know-how of correct breathing. Often teachers tend to overcomplicate the

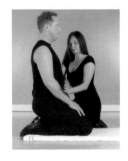

Carole helping Michael to make full use of his breathing in order to maximize his potential when performing cardiovascular, weight training and stretching exercises.

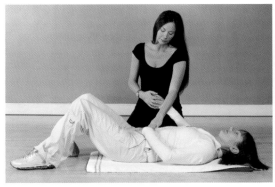
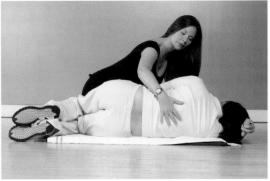

technique when in fact correct breathing is extremely simple. Have you ever watched somebody breathe while they are asleep, in particular a baby? You will notice that the whole diaphragm, torso and chest expand and then releases like an accordion. This is the complete opposite to what most of us do in our daily lives and also when we are exercising. Correct breathing applied to all movement and exercise increases capacity in every muscle, increases stamina and transforms results in mobility and flexibility, strength and stamina. See www.lifesmart.co.uk for full instructions.

(Left) Carole places one of Alison's hands on her stomach, and one on Carole's, to help her understand how and where to breathe. (Above) Carole puts Alison on her side to expand Alison's breathing into the back of her diaphragm and ribs, as well as her stomach and chest.

Posture

Make sure that you have access to a full-length mirror, then stand sideways on, taking care that this is true to how you normally stand. Let's take Alison as an example (see below). She walks with her feet turned out. Her normal stance is to over-lean into her pelvis and over-extend her neck. Her buttocks are contracted and as a result her quadriceps are tight and the base of her spine is constantly compressed causing her irritation in that area 95 per cent of the time. Her

Carole helps Alison to understand and achieve correct postural alignment.

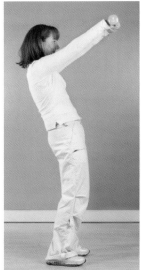
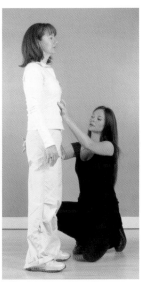
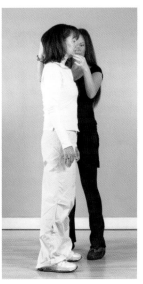

shoulders are rounded and her chest and diaphragm are slightly collapsed. As a result her pelvic floor is very weak and whereas the rest of her body is in great shape her stomach is the one area that is letting her down. Most of us, who haven't worked on our posture, have similar discrepancies. For good posture:

• Put your feet hip width apart, making sure they are facing forward and that you are fully engaging the big toe and the instep. This is often not mentioned as part of good posture but is important in engaging the adductor muscles which support the pelvic floor. People also have a tendency to roll on to the outside of their feet causing unnecessary wear and tear in other muscle groups.

• Bend your knees slightly, put the back of one hand on the base of your spine and the front of the other just under your rib cage.

• Stick your bottom out and push your shoulders back creating an arch in your spine (make sure your knees are square and not caving into each other).

• Gently push your pelvis forward, bringing your rib cage back until they are aligned in the centre and are in direct line with your hip bone. Take care not to tighten the buttocks.

• Allow your arms to drop by your side and your ribs to lift and extend fully. Your chest and thorax will open out and your shoulders will fall back and down.

• Let your chin drop down slightly so that the vertebrae in the back of your neck are in alignment with the rest of your spine and are relaxed.

• Straighten the knees without locking them out and practise your breathing for a couple of minutes in that position. By allowing the rib cage to be lifted to full potential the capacity of the diaphragm is doubled.

Try this position against a wall or lying on the floor, arching your back away from the surfaces at first, and then roll the small of your back into the surface and tilt your pelvis forward, until your whole spine and shoulder blades are touching the surfaces. Relax the buttock muscles.

Whether you are sitting on a machine, lying on a bench or standing doing weights you should emulate this position as it allows maximum potential to be gained in each muscle group with the least risk of injury. It means that the posture of your limbs will also adjust to the most correct and beneficial position. Enacting exercises in this posture is known as *still body movement*. Think of posture as a continuous stretch, constantly opening up, expanding, stabilizing and supporting all activity and movement.

Stretching

In the last couple of years there has been an improvement in knowledge about stretching in general, especially of the upper body muscle groups, but it is still undervalued and underutilized.

Each person's structure is so different, as is the muscle memory and habits of formative years, that as long as you relax into what you can do and you give the stretch the adequate amount of time and breathing, that is all your body requires

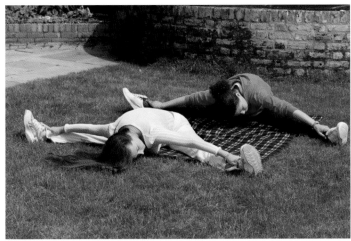

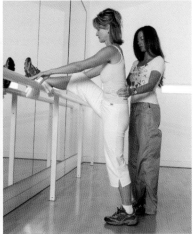

from you. If this is done consistently and the stretches are varied you will improve, most probably beyond all recognition.

What you have to watch out for, if you are very flexible, is not to overstretch the ligaments. This can happen if your regime is mainly stretch orientated and the goal of your chosen class is to turn yourself inside out. Whatever your ability, what doesn't differ is how great you will feel as a result of stretching. If any of the sitting and lying exercises prove to be difficult, you can try doing them on your bed, or with a yoga block placed under the back of your head and the base of your spine when lying down, or under your bottom if stretching in a sitting position. You will find them much easier, helping to build confidence and muscle memory.

Stretching reduces the risk of muscle soreness and injury, while increasing flexibility. Each position should be held for a minimum of 30 seconds depending on the area you are stretching and how long it takes to fully feel relaxed from the stretch. The goal is not to get to double-jointed status: feeling a bit of resistance is fine, but you shouldn't feel any pain.

Inflexibility in the back occurs in two main areas: between the shoulder blades and at the base of the spine. Stiffness in the upper back is often due to shortened muscles that occur along the arm and across the chest. For the base of the spine their partners in crime are tight hip flexors and hamstrings (back of thighs) and most importantly quadriceps that have shortened considerably, putting extra strain on the base of the spine.

Whatever regime you follow, it is useful to know the value and importance of keeping the pelvis and hips in an asymmetrical position when performing any upper or lower body stretches. Often you will see an individual stretching their hamstrings with one leg up on a bar and the standing leg turned out, twisting the pelvis and spine out of alignment. This is the body's way of cheating and it very rarely gets corrected.

(Above left) Carole and Becky doing a sitting down stretch in second position concentrating on breathing and using natural body weight and a static position to open up muscles. (Above and below) Deborah is conducting two stretches on the bar using an asymmetrical posture throughout, ensuring the pelvis and base of spine are not twisted out of alignment.

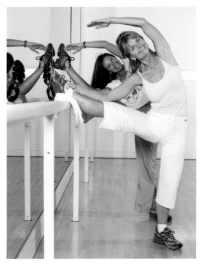

We all have one side of our body that is more flexible than the other and we automatically stretch the easier side first. Remember to spend extra time on the stiffer side and also alternate at each session which side you start on. This will promote muscle memory and equal ability on both sides of your body.

See www.lifesmart.co.uk for instructions on the bar and other stretching exercises.

A Note On Knees

It is usually considered in the gym world that the knee should always be slightly bent. Having talked to many physiotherapists and osteopaths, I find that they do not agree at all. One of the problems most people have is that they can't extend the back of their knees fully. You actually need a mix of bending and straightening of these muscles to get the right balance, engaging both the upper and lower parts of the legs. When stretching, this allows the hamstring to extend fully, which in turn strengthens the quadriceps, particularly just above the knee. It is, however, correct when standing in a static position performing upper body weight training to have slightly bent knees while your feet are parallel and hip width apart. Hyperextended joints should always maintain a slight break.

Pliés (Thigh Flexions)

The vast majority of people's bodies are not correctly aligned. Learning about your own discrepancies is a key factor. Raised hips and shoulders on one side of the body are very common, as are rotated pelvises, which can greatly impair flexibility. Often injuries that are repetitive or mysterious are a result of these physical quirks. Both strength and stamina are greatly improved by increasing flexibility and this applies equally to men as well as women.

Michael, Alison and Pearl. Different ages, different levels, problems and capabilities, all performing the plié.

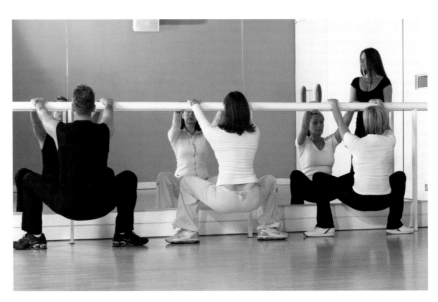

Bar exercises are designed to detect and correct any inconsistencies and build strength throughout the body for more exertive pursuits such as squats, lunges, skiing or snowboarding. The plié, or thigh flexion, will encourage you to use correct posture and breathing while doing certain isolation movements. These exercises are also bone loading, concentrating on the traction of the spine and forearms. Pliés strengthen the front of the thighs, the lateral muscles and trapezius (upper back) at the same time as stretching the inner thigh muscles. Pliés can also be done with the feet slightly closer together on half point, making sure that you take equal weight on the little toe as well as the big toe and further work the strength and range of motion in the feet and the calves, the pelvic floor, knees and thighs – particularly on rising from plié to standing position.

Inflexibility coupled with misalignment can be responsible for many mysterious and repetitive strain injuries, so as a foundation for all men and women the bar exercises in particular are important.

When men do these exercises, they cannot believe how much they sweat. Women who consider themselves to be very athletic and strong are also surprised at the intensity they experience when doing pliés. In effect what you are doing is activating the lymph and blood flow throughout every part of your body. Performing cardiovascular exercise or weights after doing bar exercises takes on a completely different feel and result.

See www.lifesmart.co.uk for full instructions.

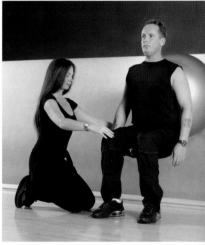

Ball wall squat. An excellent way to work quads, hamstrings, and gluts. Carole is making sure that Michael's vertebrae position, knees, ankles and feet are asymmetrical, and correct.

Exercise Balls

Originally used as a tool for rehabilitation, the exercise ball, usually 55, 65 or 75 centimetres in diameter, defies its seemingly basic appearance to be an incredibly effective piece of exercise equipment, bringing muscles into play that traditional weight training cannot. It is used for core training, which is best achieved when the body is placed in an unstable environment as it forces the core muscles to stabilize the body while working deeper layers of muscles. Other equipment that can also be used for this kind of training are wobble boards and foam rollers.

(Left and below) Michael using the exercise ball to improve upper body flexibility.

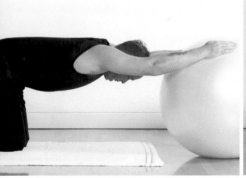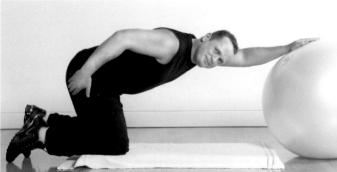

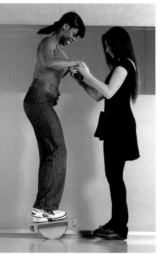

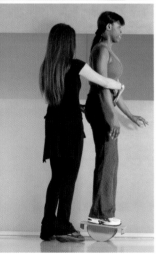

Jocelyn on the wobble board. Being supremely fit, she had seldom worked on core stability before, and she found it almost impossible to begin with – but eventually mastered it!

Exercise balls can help improve posture, which in turn decreases stress to the joints and stabilizes muscles. They can improve your balance and stability by working the neutralizer and stabilizer muscles and they are also good for stretching and spine alignment. They can be used with body weight alone or in conjunction with machines and free weights.

If you find it hard at the beginning – and exercise balls are a lot harder to use than they look – please don't give up. It takes time to develop the balance required to use the equipment correctly, and it's not just about preventing you from falling off – proper positioning must be maintained throughout. The pelvis needs to be tucked in and the belly button pulled into the back without tightening the buttocks. I wouldn't recommend using this apparatus without first receiving guidance from a qualified trainer.

Core Stability

Most people focus their attention on the more visible and easy-to-train muscles such as the pectorals (chest) and biceps (front of upper arm) but overlook the most important muscles that act as our foundation. Core stability refers to the small, deep lumbar spine and trunk muscles (the inner muscles that make up the abdominal region, hips and lower back) and the supportive effect they have on the area – or, as Joseph Pilates described it, the 'girdle of strength'. These muscles are not involved in producing the movements – they use static or isometric contractions – but they are required to hold the lumbar spine in its correct alignment nearly continuously, not only during exercise but throughout everyday activities.

The functional result of good core stability is shown when an athlete is performing a sporting movement and is able to maintain the correct posture and alignment. An improved technique will help to reduce injury risk. Good examples are diving and gymnastic events.

The first step is to learn how to achieve a 'neutral' lumbar position and perform hollowing exercises, which you will find at www.lifesmart.co.uk.

Abdominal Muscles

Cutting back on dietary fat and having a trim waist does not necessarily mean you have a toned stomach; there is a difference between strengthening the abdominal area and reducing your body fat. But if you follow a healthy eating regime and perform abdominal exercises to strengthen the area you will eventually develop a strong and toned stomach!

Side bends are an important element of working the core area, toning and strengthening the abdominal obliques (love handles) and spinal muscles and stimulating the main organs, for example the liver, kidneys, stomach and spleen. There are many exercises you can use to work this area, either standing or lying on the floor or using an exercise ball.

The mistake people often make is in trying to 'spot reduce' fat bulges from the sides of their waist by overdoing side bends and twists with weights that are too heavy, coupled with too many repetitions. This overloads the obliques and makes the bulges worse by building up the muscle beneath the fat layer. When performing this exercise make sure you utilize correct posture and maintain an asymmetrical position throughout your torso. Use pulsing with no weights and only slow, continuous, controlled movement when using a weight. Make the stretch element and correct pelvic position of primary importance in both cases.

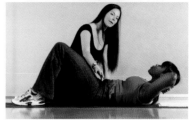

Pelvic Floor Exercises

Pelvic floor or Kegel exercises (named after the American gynaecologist Dr Arnold Kegel), target the pelvic floor, which supports the bladder and bowel. The pelvic floor is made up of layers of muscle resembling a hammock which stretches from the tailbone at the back to the pubic bone in the front and forms the body's 'undercarriage'.

(Above and below) A variety of exercises for core stability, pelvic floor and stomachs. Go to www.lifesmart.co.uk for the full range of these and other relevant exercises.

Its many roles are to support the pelvic organs and abdominal contents, help to hold the bladder, womb and bowel in place and to control the muscles that close the anus, vagina and urethra. The muscles can be weakened by childbirth; continual straining to empty your bowels, usually due to constipation; a chronic cough, such as smoker's cough; chronic bronchitis or asthma; heavy lifting; neurological damage, for example after a stroke or spinal injury; and obesity.

When the pelvic floor muscles are weakened or damaged this can result in stress incontinence, decreased satisfaction during intercourse and prolapses. The good news is that like most muscles they can be strengthened with exercise.

These exercises have for years been considered the domain of women only, in particular throughout pregnancy and during and after childbirth. Strong pelvic floor muscles can support the extra weight of pregnancy, help in the second stage of labour, and, by increasing your circulation, assist after birth in healing

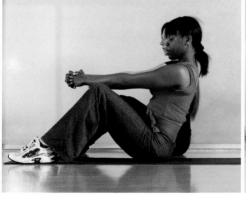

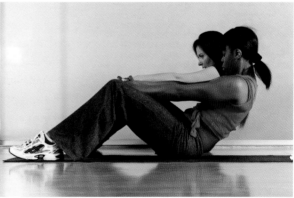

the perineum, which is between the anus and vagina. Now, it has been proven that men suffering from erectile dysfunction can also benefit greatly from maintaining the muscle tone and function of their pelvic floors.

According to the Impotence Association, the exercises strengthen the muscles around the penis, improving the blood supply to the pelvis and thus 'enhance orgasmic sensations by strengthening the pelvic muscles that produce ejaculation by their contraction'. It's even being said that doing these simple exercises can result in the same success as taking Viagra. Any healthy and natural alternative to drugs is in my opinion something that can not be encouraged enough.

Obviously, feeling confident that you are exercising the correct muscles is of vital importance. Like a child learning to wink without using all his facial muscles, learning to isolate the pelvic floor, while refraining from clenching the buttocks, contracting the stomach and holding your breath can be tricky, but like anything new the more you practise the easier it becomes.

I remember the first time I had to teach pelvic floor exercises to a room full of fellow students. Of course there were the usual red faces and giggling when it came to the anus and vagina! I was lucky, however, to receive sound advice from one of the instructors. He simply said that if I showed embarrassment at teaching the exercise then how did I think my clients would feel? He emphasized that I needed to accept the importance of teaching pelvic floor exercises as an integral part of my training sessions.

To this day I am grateful for his down-to-earth attitude. I passed the exam without even getting embarrassed and since then I've refused to let either myself or my clients feel any embarrassment. However, I do tell them that they don't have to look me in the eye while doing the exercise!

One of the best ways of locating the muscles is to divide and conquer. Starting with the vagina/penis, while passing water, attempt to stop the flow of urine. If you can do this then you have successfully located the forward muscle. However, do not do this on a regular basis as it can cause urinary infections.

Nearly everyone has felt the need at one time or another to pass wind at a very inconvenient time and has held it in by squeezing the anus closed tight, creating a 'pulling' feeling. If you can do this then you have successfully located the second muscle.

I describe to my clients the muscle looking like a hammock with two sets of elevator doors, one at each end. I ask them to close the doors at the front (vagina), and while keeping them closed to then close the doors at the back (anus). Once the doors are closed tightly we start to ascend and, as I count from one to five each number is a separate floor. Once we reach the top we slowly descend to the ground floor where we stop and pause. It is imperative that the muscles are not released quickly, but that they are controlled and released in a slow manner and you have a definite feeling of letting go.

Working the muscles quickly is also essential in helping them react to sudden stresses from coughing, laughing or exercise that puts pressure on the bladder. So by practising quick contractions you are prepared for any emergency. This time squeeze both doors closed and up at the same time, holding for one second, before releasing them slowly down. Try and increase the time you hold the contraction, building up to 10 seconds. This is known as 'squeeze until you sneeze', and once you have developed strong muscles you will have far fewer accidents.

You can alternate the exercises, and for optimum results try to do them around 50 to 100 times a day. To safeguard against problems recurring you should maintain the exercises on a daily basis.

It is impossible to see someone performing pelvic floor exercises as they take place internally and can be done while lying down, sitting or standing. Try and get into the habit of doing them while stuck at red traffic lights, when you're doing the washing up, in a queue at the bank, post office or supermarket and even during meetings with your boss. My only warning is that some people have been known to curl their toes or raise their eyebrows in time with the lifts and that alone might cause some funny looks!

Weight Training
Weight training builds muscle mass and large muscles burn more calories than smaller ones, so the simple equation is 'more muscle equals more fat burned'. Bulking need not be a prerequisite, as long as you balance everything with stretching and are sensible about the load you are using. Women do not have the genetic disposition to bulk up like men, unless you have been very active in certain areas of sport where you have built considerable muscle mass or you are naturally built that way. If that is the case, make sure that you maintain a balance by using your own body as resistance mixed with stretches and light to moderate weights.

Joints And Upper And Lower Body Resistance Training
The stability of your joints is essential to minimize injury, but commonly they are subject to misplacement in both upper and lower body weight and resistance training. Whether you are using a machine, free weights or your own body

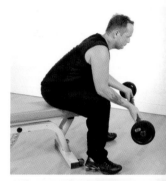
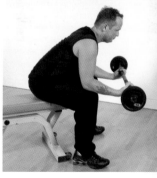

Lower arm and wrist strengthening exercise. Michael's forearms are resting on his thighs whilst his back is fully extended and straight, chest lifted and shoulders away from the ears.

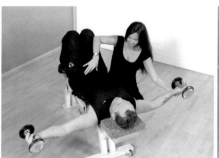
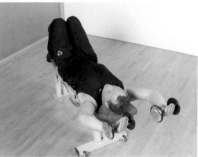

(Left) Michael uses two light weights to open up and expand his chest muscles whilst anchoring the pelvic floor to share the distribution of weight.

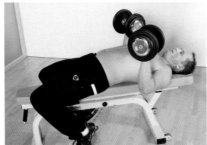 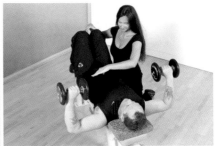

(Right) Incorrect leg position and execution of chest press. Any number of injuries can occur. (Far right) Correct position and execution of chest press.

resistance, the alignment of your limbs should be asymmetric. This means your knees should never go over your toes when doing lunges and squats, and your elbows should remain in line with your wrists and shoulder joints when performing chest, shoulder, bicep and tricep exercises.

When it comes to the wrists it's also important to check that they are in the right position. Any extreme postures, such as extended wrists (bent backwards), often used during bicep curls or chest presses, must be avoided as they can cause increased stress to the joints between the carpal bones and increased tension to the tendons crossing the wrist. Whenever possible, try to keep the wrists straight during activity. Using resistance machines and performing free weights using both hands and arms in unison helps to at first distribute the load and results in increased control of the wrist position. This also allows you to concentrate on establishing perfect posture while executing the different actions maintaining a still body position. Alternate moves can be used once you are confident and strong enough.

Upper Body – Sitting And Lying Postures

Resistance machine chest press. The posture of all limbs is as important as the posture of the spine.

Whether you are using a resistance machine or free weights' bench, how you sit and lie is of equal importance to how you stand. You want to avoid being hunched or arching your back away from the chair. So press your spine and shoulder blades into the chair, ensure your rib cage is fully expanded, allowing your chest to be fully open with your shoulders back and relaxed without arching your back away from the seat.

To ensure the top of the vertebrae is tension-free, as well as stabilizing the head and neck, allow the chin to drop slightly (some people have a tendency to push their head and shoulders away from the chair in order to help push a heavy weight). If you are sitting on a resistance machine put your feet firmly on the floor either side of the machine's foot pad as Pearl is doing on the chest-press machine (see left). Gently press the feet into the floor, tilting the pelvis at the same time, thus activating all the lower body muscles to give you extra stability and support. Hold your stomach muscles in a contracted position.

Assume the same position when doing a free weights chest press on a bench as Michael is doing with the dumbbells (see above). If you are lying down, rest your feet on the opposite end of the bench to your head so that you can fully engage

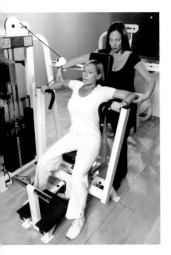

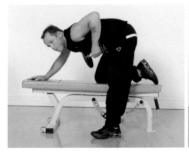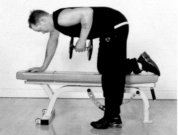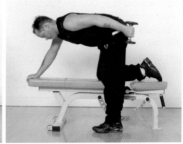

your pelvic floor and stomach muscles for extra support. Put a block under your head if there is too much of a gap between your neck and the bench. This will allow your chin to tilt slightly forward in order for your upper vertebrae to be straight.

Dumbbell kickbacks. (Above left) A commonly executed incorrect position. (Centre and above) Michael is demonstrating correct posture and fixed upper arm position, crucial to this exercise.

Upper Body – Standing

When standing to perform free-weight training of the upper body, the legs should be facing forward, feet straight and hip width apart, the knees slightly bent, the pelvis gently tilted without tightening the buttocks, the stomach contracted, diaphragm lifted, shoulders back and down and the chin slightly dropped. If the exercise is particularly challenging, place one foot in front of the other, still keeping a hip width between the feet.

(Below) Cable pulldown. (Bottom) Remedial rotator cuff strengthener.

Triceps – Dumbbell Kickbacks

Most people perform this exercise and the one-arm dumbbell row in an incorrect position. They have a hunched back, their knees are too far forward under them and they use momentum to service a too-heavy weight with the movement performed over too big a range. See Michael's incorrect and correct positions.

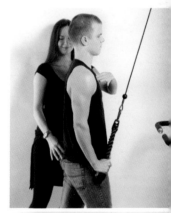

Triceps – Cable Pulldown

This is one of the classic exercises that we often see being done incorrectly, especially by men. They pile on the weights and stand in an ape-like position, demonstrating momentum at its best or worst, depending on how you look at it!

Nothing can show you the need for a still body technique better than the cable pulldown.

Wrist Curls

The wrists and extensor muscles in the lower arms are often overlooked and end up being weak. An excellent exercise for strengthening these areas is wrist curls. See the exercise on page 157.

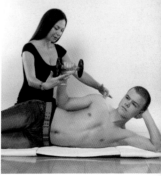

Rotator Cuff

The rotator cuff comprises a group of tendons and muscles that attach the bone of the upper arm to the shoulder blade, providing support and mobility to the ball-and-socket joint of the shoulder. There is an important connection between the pectoral and deltoid muscles because of the overlap of various muscle groups at the point of insertion. If they aren't suitably stretched there is a notable contraction which can result in the shoulders rotating forward which in turn will overthrow the whole muscular skeletal frame, adversely affecting both the chest area and spine.

A common reason for shoulder pain is a rotator cuff tear, which can result from a single traumatic incident or develop from repetitive activities, such as painting a ceiling, heavy lifting or simply the reduction of blood to the tendon due to ageing.

A few of the signs are constant pain, particularly when carrying out overhead movements, muscle weakness when lifting the arm, limited mobility, and most commonly an unpleasant clicking sensation when making ordinary everyday movements. This can be prevented or treated by resting the shoulder from overuse, postural changes and remedial exercises. See the exercise on page 159.

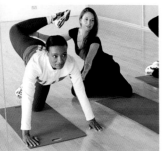

(Below) Audrey demonstrates a hip flexor mobility and isolation exercise.

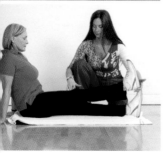

(Above) Thigh and knee strengthening exercise. (Below) Incorrect and correct positions for a single leg squat.

Lower Body

There is as much choice of standing floor exercises and mat work for lower body work as there are machines and apparatus. The advantage is that you can work very precisely on any given area and on the remedial aspects to stiff hip flexors, shortened quadriceps or tight limbs as well as toning, balance and core stability.

For example, to knit the upper body and lower body together, without the use of machines, hip flexor exercises on all fours utilizing upper body strength by holding the position while increasing hip flexor mobility, are among the toughest exercises anyone can do. If you are consistent this will make all the difference as you age, as it will help to prevent hip and back problems.

Lower Body Machines

Often I watch people whose posture and feet are limp when using these machines. The results and improvements are slow or non-existent. Correct

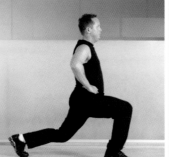
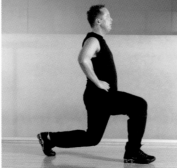
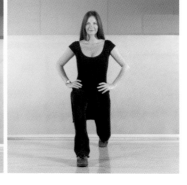

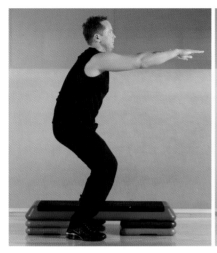
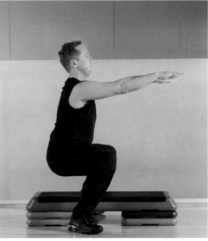

The squat. (Far left) Michael's shoulders are tense and hunched, and his spine is curved. A common sight but incorrect.
(Left) His spine is straight, shoulders are relaxed and away from his ears.

upper body posture, as described, while engaging your core muscles makes a huge difference to the safety and outcome of this exercise. On the lower body, the key component is always to flex the feet which immediately activates the other leg muscles. The power, support and control come directly from positioning your feet in this way. Always remember to do as full a movement as possible and perform it slowly for best results. Never snap the knees straight, and whatever the resistance machine, when releasing the legs to starting position throughout repetitions, don't release the weight completely until the last movement is performed.

At www.lifesmart.co.uk you can access a starter pack of exercises including all the ones mentioned in this chapter.

Yoga

Consuelo Fernandez Andia was born in Chile in 1953 and moved to London in 1974 where she has been practising yoga for the past 30 years. She has an International Yoga Certificate and is also a qualified Sports Massage Therapist, teaching in health clubs and in schools where she educates both children and teachers. Consuelo describes yoga as a 'sculptor of the body, mind and soul'.

Since aerobics and weight training have become so popular, yoga has been the subject of some criticism. As with every activity it has its dangers – particularly if a teacher has a large ego and insists on elaborate poses or pushing your flexibility beyond its boundaries. You need a teacher who can get to know each person in the class and their limits. Many people worldwide have gained remarkable benefits from yoga, which not only include increased flexibility, but also for some a spiritual awareness and self-esteem. Others have transformed their shape, and for most a sense of calm has been achieved.

Correct breathing is the tool for a very rewarding journey through yoga. As Consuelo explains, there are two main functions of proper breathing: the first is

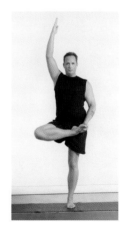

This yoga position strengthens and firms legs, improving physical and mental poise.

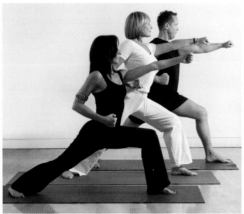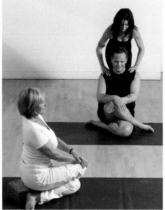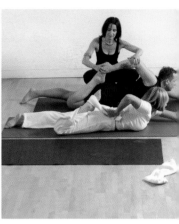

(Above) Warrior pose. This generates strength, vigour and courage. (Centre) A difficult but wonderful hip opener which strengthens the back and encourages concentration. (Far right) Bow posture – the whole front of the body is stretched and firmed, the stomach muscles are massaged and the abdominal viscera stimulated and toned.

to bring more oxygen to the blood and therefore to the brain; the second is to control the vital life energy. Yoga consists of a series of exercises especially intended to meet these needs and keep the body in vibrant health. The beauty of yoga is its pure simplicity. You do not need to be an acrobat, an athlete or have a fantastic body shape; you just need to be yourself.

Pilates

Joseph H. Pilates was born in Düsseldorf, Germany in 1880. His childhood was plagued by rickets, asthma and rheumatic fever, and yearning for a healthy, strong, physically attractive body his interest in body conditioning started at an early age. He read copious amounts on everything from anatomy to yoga, Zen meditation to ancient Greek and Roman exercise regimes.

In 1912 he left Germany to train as a boxer in England where, during World War One, he worked as a nurse helping patients immobilized by war injuries. Pilates eventually developed his own method of 500 controlled exercises focused on developing 'core' muscles of the abdomen and increased flexibility in the arms, legs and supporting muscle groups.

He believed in 'complete coordination of body, mind and spirit' and his regime stressed quality of movement over quantity of repetitions, resulting in a body that was strong and sleek with a natural grace.

From England, he emigrated to the United States, where in 1926 he opened the Pilates Studio. Since then, his system has been used by individuals at all fitness levels, as well as by dance companies, sports teams and fitness enthusiasts. Pilates continued to develop his technique and teach in his studio until his death in 1967.

Stephanie Beeson, one of England's top Pilates teachers, has studied anatomy, dance and Pilates and continues to research biomechanics and apply it to her Pilates work. Her background has been diverse, studying with instructors in New York, London and Geneva. There are very few teachers in England who have Stephanie's level of accuracy and expertise. Having done Pilates in the UK, US

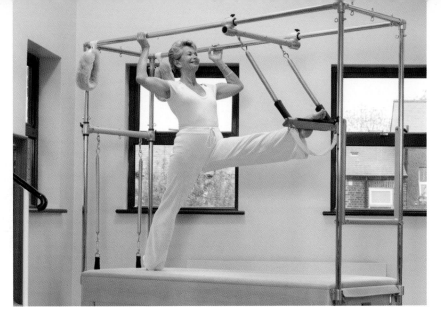

and Australia, I can honestly say that many forms of Pilates taught in the UK are unrecognizable to that taught by the masters. However, that doesn't mean you won't derive benefits from them.

Joseph Pilates never prescribed exactly how his method should be taught, and therefore Pilates is taught in many different ways. The methods he developed for a boxer were very different from those designed for a dentist or a dancer, making it difficult for people to know who is teaching the 'real' system. For some the 'real' system only includes the choreography of the classical exercises as taught in the studio on the Pilates equipment, while for others it is more about the detail in how the movements should be performed.

Stephanie believes that a 'real' Pilates teacher should be able to do both, knowing the full choreography and the detail and they should have the skills to safely take someone from the core principles through to the classical choreography.

It is difficult for the public to know the difference between someone who teaches 'Pilates-based' classes from 'Pilates' classes. 'Pilates-based' usually means they focus on core stability but are not teaching the original 'classical' exercises. It often also implies an instructor who has taken a Pilates workshop but has not undergone a comprehensive training programme. Many instructors are calling their classes Pilates when they are really teaching pre-Pilates exercises. Pre-Pilates exercises focus on the basic elements of the system but the instructor is often not comprehensively trained in the full repertoire of mat exercises.

Proper Pilates instructors have to learn in a studio for at least two years before starting out on their own. Now people can learn the system in modular form. Most start with training to teach the mat work, which is problematic if they stop there and think they know the whole system. The complete system utilizes movements performed on Pilates-based equipment (spring) to help people develop the skills they need to perform the mat exercises unaided. When someone only knows the mat techniques they often have gaps in their knowledge of how they use their own bodies. To teach Pilates you must know the system in your own body. You wouldn't teach French if you couldn't speak it, yet there are many calling themselves 'Pilates' teachers who only know 'phrases' from the system and are far from 'fluent'.

Comprehensively trained Pilates teachers will be able to look at you performing a movement and guide your bones into the correct alignment. Instructors must also understand what an aligned body looks like in all positions. They should be able to 'see' a joint that is not centered and have the skill to help their clients develop the sensory awareness to know what centered alignment feels like. Detailed knowledge of the musculo-skeletal system is essential, with good knowledge of the joints and which muscles act to stabilize them.

Basic principles should include breathing, the ability to curl the head off the floor without overworking the muscles at the front of the neck, movement of the thigh or arm without disturbing the stability of the pelvis or shoulder, and the core stability of the torso.

Pilates focuses on core stability but also stability for the whole body while moving. There is a very big difference. It's not just what you are doing that is important but the way you are doing it that makes a movement a Pilates exercise.

Currently there are no national standards for Pilates teachers in the UK. The US-based Pilates Method Alliance is the only independent organization offering advice about Pilates, see www.pilatesmethodalliance.org. All other associations are private and commercially run and will only list teachers they have trained. See also www.pilatesfoundation.co.uk and Stephanie@enavantpilates.fsnet.co.uk

Abdominal Muscles

The way in which Pilates trains your abdominal muscles (abs) is one of the reasons for its popularity. The key is to engage your transverses or deepest abdominal layer in readiness for any movement you make. This hollowing from the navel to the spine supports your pelvis and lower back, keeping it safe. Pilates as a system focuses on this core strength and many of the exercises work directly by challenging the power once it has been found. Often just waking up this area is the first challenge! A common mistake is not getting the bones in the right place. This means addressing the alignment of the head, ribs and pelvis before targeting the abs. This is where a Pilates teacher is invaluable: we ourselves often have difficulty sensing where we are and a less than ideal alignment often feels 'normal'.

Men And Pilates

The focus on the stabilizing muscles of the skeleton creates a strong base of support, enabling the larger more powerful moving muscles to work more efficiently and

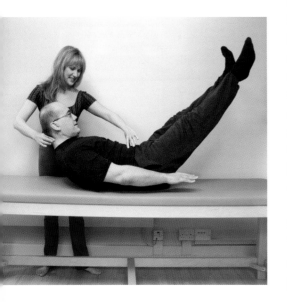

The 100s is a classical mat exercise in Pilates. Imprinting the spine, not 'tucking' the pelvis, ensures the back is supported against the weight of the legs. It wakes up the abdominals, legs and arms ready for a Pilates session. Start with a count of 20 (inhaling for a count of 5 and exhaling for a count of 5), increasing by 5 until you reach 100.

often with greater power. It is easy to spend more time on the larger muscles, but this can lead to imbalances which can result in injury. Muscle balance is part of the Pilates system and this includes freedom of movement or flexibility. Flexibility is often missing from men's workout programmes. Using the Pilates equipment enables you to balance your strength with flexibility. The springs can rest already powerful muscles giving the chance for the stability muscles to kick in. Pilates is a great cross-training system to support other sports and activities. It keeps you fit and protects you from injury so that you can enjoy other activities.

Kickboxing

Keith Wilson has been a professional kickboxer and personal trainer since 1985 and has held British and European championship titles in kickboxing. He began by studying Wado Ryu Karate, reaching 1st degree black belt by the age of 19. He has trained and competed in boxing, recording 21 amateur contests over a three-year period before turning to kickboxing where he reached the rank of 5th degree (Dan) black belt.

Boxing-style workouts help to develop strength, endurance, mobility and suppleness. Reflexes are sharpened and the body naturally reacts faster according to the situation, be it in a gym environment or in the unfortunate situation of being physically threatened.

From the first session it is imperative that the coach instils the correct stance and foot positioning. I first started working with Keith 10 years ago before boxing was brought into the gym environment. From Keith's travels he is aware of how many personal trainers, with limited experience in the fundamentals of boxing training, are simply holding up a pair of pads and allowing their clients to flail away aimlessly in order to achieve some kind of aerobic/anaerobic respiratory distress and perhaps release some stress – which in itself is no bad thing. However, correct technique is vital and should not be omitted for the sake of aerobic benefit or to provide variety to an individual's workout routine.

Some health clubs hold one- or two-day courses in setting up a form of boxercise regime. This is where the problem lies. A coach can't be made competent in just a couple of days – you need to have a good basic knowledge and experience. The club trainers are aware of how the body works, how to maintain body fat levels, develop lean body mass and get people in good shape. What is worrying though is the way they are coaching kickboxing and boxing. Unfortunately, people are sacrificing good positioning and aren't holding their hands up defensively, their chin is too high, and their elbows are too far out. This means that the number one rule for protecting your most vulnerable parts (i.e. your face and ribs) is not being followed. On top of that, incorrect body posture results in poor stability, jagged movements and impaired aim.

Carole delivers a roundhouse kick. A powerful whipping kick using the body's rotation and sudden twisting of the support leg and hip.

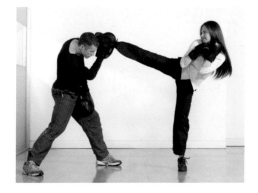

Boxing is a complex routine which should be constantly built on – especially if you are to enter into combat. Keith has seen untrained people enter the ring, often with disastrous consequences. However, there are properly trained kickboxing or boxing instructors around – you just need to take the trouble to seek them out.

Boxing may be used as a cross-training component and may be integrated with other enjoyable activities, such as yoga, running, swimming, cycling, resistance and strength training; in fact anything which works on conditioning the body will supplement a boxing/kickboxing regime. For example, a marathon runner or triathlete working on endurance might want to break up the monotony of mileage by incorporating a boxing workout fortnightly. This will strengthen the upper body and trunk muscles, and help increase physical and mental strength.

Basic punching techniques are initially delivered simply against the air before hitting against a padded target. Wearing boxing gloves, you hit focus pads held by your trainer, developing the ability to throw various punches while developing power in your body. Optional kicking techniques are introduced allowing the practitioner to develop the strong kicks from the kickboxer's repertoire.

Use of elbow and knee striking techniques are introduced at the trainer's discretion, enabling powerful blows to be delivered at close range in a defensive situation. Eventually moving on to sparring, shadowboxing, parrying, blocking, evasive slipping, ducking foot work, jabs, right crosses, left hooks etc. Workouts can last anywhere between 30 and 90 minutes, but on average last one hour.

Right upper cut. An explosive close range punch delivered upwards with the power coming from the right foot up through the right hip and out through the right fist – palm towards body on impact. The right foot should be firmly planted on impact, again dipping at the knees on delivery.

Punches

Punches should travel through space in a fast yet relaxed fashion, explode on the target, pass several inches through the target, snap back along the same pathway travelled, and end up with the fist in its defensive position next to the face.

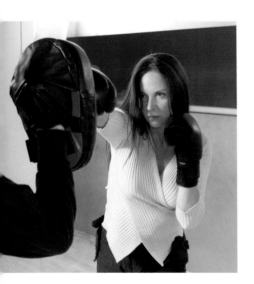

Basic punches must be learnt individually and correctly before moving on to basic combination punches. Remember that the power for all punches commences at the ground so the feet should be firmly planted on delivery, otherwise power will be dissipated and loss of balance could occur.

In addition it is important that one is well-protected while throwing punches or launching an attack, for example, the non-punching hand should be up, the chin down and the elbows in, as in real combat there could well be incoming punches.

Tips

• All punches should be delivered with the outside three knuckles of the fist hitting the target. Be careful not to land solely with the little finger as it is weak and can easily be damaged.

• You should exhale on the delivery of the punch; the breathing in part will take care of itself after a lifetime of practise!

• When carrying out an upper cut do not drop the punching hand too far, rather dip the body and bring the hand explosively upwards while dipping.

• When throwing any punch the opposite hand should always be pressed to the side of the face.

• It is important to return a movement along the same pathway as the delivery.

• A combat situation is extremely stressful, so it is important to always practise the movements correctly in addition to keeping the body relaxed, without locked joints. This will make the movements flow instinctively, so they become second nature to the combatant, not stiff or wooden.

• As you develop, you should work on moving after throwing punches, becoming a moving target yourself as opposed to standing still. Parrying and evasive moves are learned, as well as how to get up on the toes and move rapidly and laterally away from one's opponent.

• Remember: keeping small will keep you better protected.

Equipment

You will need the following:

• Hand wraps; weighted boxing gloves (depending on body weight and hand size); light, flat-soled boots (for ankle support); non-restrictive clothing.

• Wearing of hand wraps and correct fitting boxing type gloves will ensure minimal injuries to the hands and wrists.

For more information on Keith Wilson and Albany Kickboxing see www.albanykickboxing.com. For details of all the exercises in this chapter see www.lifesmart.co.uk.

Conclusion

Exercise should be contagious as opposed to an effort. All you have to do is start somewhere that is simple and without too much pressure. Book a massage as a reward for your first week of physical pursuits. Go for the enjoyment that using and feeling your body results in. There is no right time, as the apathy of the mind usually outweighs all good intentions and reasons. As the saying so aptly goes: 'Use it or lose it!'.

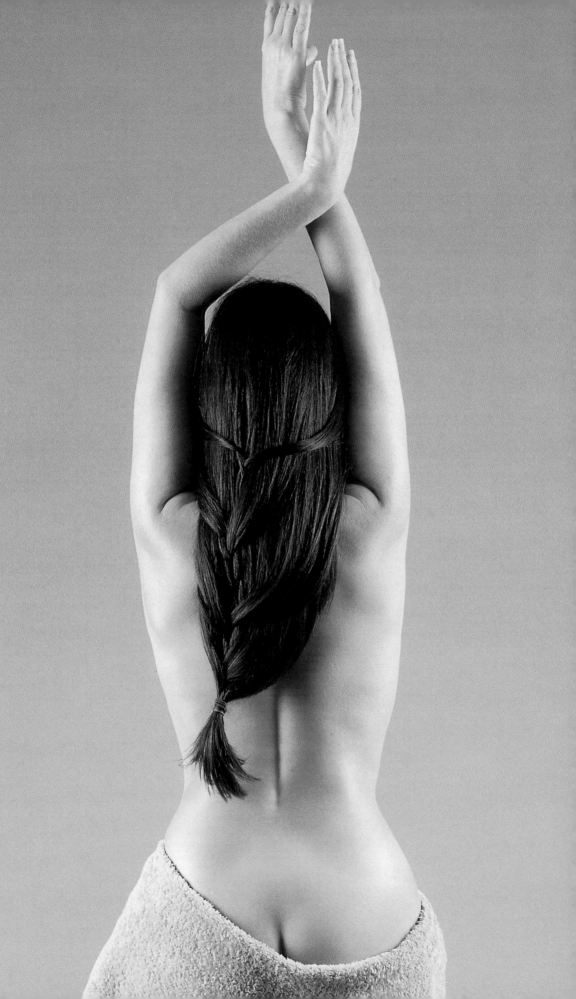

DESSERTS
USE YOUR IDEAS

Taking Care

TAKING CARE OF YOURSELF is often seen as frivolous, female-only territory. Thankfully, that is changing. But what does it mean to really take care of yourself?

Is taking care slapping on a face mask once a week? Having multiple medications at home and at work for any ailment that occurs? Going to a spa a couple of times a year and learning to '*omm*' with the best of them? Somehow I don't think so.

Mainly, taking care is all about setting up good, strong support systems to help you deal as effectively as possible with life's stresses and strains. The busier you are, the more important it is to look after yourself. In First Aid training, the number one rule is that unless you are completely safe and taken care of first, you will be of no use to anyone or will put yourself and others in jeopardy. Life is no different...

Taking care is of equal importance to men, women and children alike. For all the articles and advertisements promoting fabulous products, spas and retreats, when I look around I see a world of people who seem to have lost their way where well-being is concerned, and have put their health low on their list of priorities. In 2003, 27 million prescriptions for antidepressants were issued in the UK. Time to get a grip, don't you think?

The areas that we have to take care of, in a far more intelligent and proactive way than the majority of us do, are as follows:

• Our emotional state first and foremost. Even while asleep (and of course in daily life), we are affected by our emotions, and they can undermine every aspect of our life.

• Our environment. All the elements that are destroying our environment are also what are destroying our bodies' ability to perform in the way that we would ideally like them to. It shows up physically in the increase in low sperm counts, cancer, diabetes, heart attacks and the need for IVF treatment ... by now, you know the rest.

• Our physical bodies. You need to take care of your physical state so that you have the energy and stamina to deal with the demands of relationships, children, working and socializing. When I started doing this work, it became clear that establishing and maintaining order in people's homes made all the difference to their continuity and enthusiasm. Exhaustion is such a common problem that no matter what fabulous advice is given on food and fitness, this has to be tackled for anyone to progress. Knowledge about relaxation, sleeping, bathing and any remedial therapy such as massage or Reiki that can give you a speedy turnaround when you are feeling below par is essential. This in turn means not resorting to doctors and drugs every time your back goes or you have minor ailments, but learning how to read and naturally treat your own body. Recuperating properly when you are ill and under stress, and utilizing complementary medicine completes this package.

Structure And Boundaries

You need to have boundaries, as without this stable outline your structure will crumble before you've even begun.

For some reason the word 'boundaries' has the same stigma as rules and regulations. Yet when you look at any breakdown you've suffered, whether it be in a relationship, energy levels or even depression, the missing ingredient is so often a healthy set of boundaries.

No matter how hard it may seem to establish boundaries in your home, around your health, in your relationships and with your children, they will always end up being your best friend. Why? Because they allow you to set parameters that stop you from pushing yourself and others too far, and they demand communication and listening to take place (still a problem today in both working and personal relationships) in order to be fully successful and supportive.

When the going gets tough, the standards and structure you set up at home will mean you always have a safe haven when life deals you its inevitable blows.

Achieving Daily Equilibrium

Life happens in waves. People, work, matters of the heart and life in general all seem to be chugging along comfortably – then a wave comes in and knocks you over and it's hard not to be carried along by the current. It's at these times in particular that you need to draw on different tools to help you manage. For many people – men as well as women – it's giving yourself the time and permission to make space to digest the day or week; to write, talk, sleep and if necessary have a good cry, instead of bulldozing through life in your usual fashion. That way, you have a decent chance of coming out the other side more knowledgeable and intact as a result.

Let me explain further. When you go about your daily routine, other people's moods, behaviour and problems – especially if they are offloading on you – and even your own reactions and denials to events, leaves a residue. Whether you get a buzz from these situations or you feel drained, depressed or upset, your emotions and physical body take the brunt. This is particularly pertinent to people working in service industries, such as health practitioners, teachers, lawyers and human resources staff.

Emotional reactions are inevitable and the effects accumulate if they aren't cleared, which is often why we perpetuate or can't break harmful patterns in our lives. Meditation, visualization, self-hypnosis and breathing exercise techniques are particularly helpful here. Their purpose is to help you ground yourself, move through reactions, eradicate the negative energy left by people and events that have affected you emotionally and physically and restore your equilibrium. It's not about believing or disbelieving, rather it's to aid you in developing stability, strength and self-awareness in times of need.

In my experience, there are two types of outcome from meditation. One is where you spin off into dreamland and then eventually come back to consciousness. For some people that is enough. Other people – particularly those who experience a steady flow of ups and downs, challenges and emotions – need what I call a working meditation that is not reliant on a cult, person or even a sound. The idea is that this kind of meditation can be done anywhere, at any time, taking between five and 20 minutes. The purpose is to move you through your reaction to a perceived crisis or problem as quickly as possible as well as accessing insights and answers. By developing this discipline, your whole outlook during and after an unpleasant interlude will completely change.

Anyone who knows me will tell you that I'm not keen on 'omming' or meditating for hours. But meditation is a tool that can be quite profound in its simplicity, and it certainly beats bearing the brunt of adverse or challenging situations. There isn't any one definitive technique and you don't have to be spiritual, religious or strange to adopt any one of them.

Coming To Emotional Blows

Losing a loved one through death or through a parting of the ways is guaranteed to knock you sideways in a way that nothing else comes close to. It's at these times that I really appeal to people to be as kind as they possibly can be to themselves. Sometimes we have to be reminded that it's acceptable to bleed, it's part of the recovery process, and every area of natural self-help and nurturing throughout this book can be applied, depending on what your needs are. This is one time when the body really does want to crash and sleep and initially it shouldn't be forced into trying to do otherwise.

There is a natural cycle to grief in terms of timing. The first three days to three weeks are the most crucial period where the wound remains raw and whatever good advice or encouragement people might give often serves only to irritate and make things worse. If you find you are really sinking, the new Ainsworth Rescue Remedy and Flower Essences (see page 210), as well as homeopathic support, are excellent. Writing about any unexpressed thoughts and emotions can also be very cathartic.

During this initial period, the body is very shaky and fragile physically, and often people may experience shivering, drops in temperature, nausea, palpitations and loss of appetite. It's imperative not to rely on caffeine and alcohol at this time. Often people will punish themselves by smoking, drinking and/or drug-taking, and that's a spiral you don't want to get into.

Even if you are normally a meditator and/or user of complementary practices, it's fine if you don't feel like drawing on any of these during this time. After the first 21 days, though, whatever your reaction, there is a slight but marked shift where equilibrium begins to return.

For some people, the devastation and distortion that can arise out of grief or the break-up of a relationship means that they need some help and guidance. To hurt and rage past a certain degree can often denote unhealthy choices and patterns. Rather than slide down into low self-esteem and perceived victimhood, this is the perfect opportunity to do some necessary work on yourself.

If you go through the grieving process in a way that is as healthy and right for you as possible, three months down the line – even when you get that knot in your stomach at the thought or reminder of your loss – there is a quiet acceptance and different strength. That is what is important to build on.

Different Qualities Of Pain

Pain is the way that the body tells you it is out of balance, and sometimes you need to listen to, rather than suppress, that message. As soon as headache symptoms arise for instance, we usually suppress them through analgesic medication. Through the overuse of suppressor drugs, promoted by pharmaceutical companies, people have lost the ability to describe their pain or locate the root cause and site. Pain at the back of the head, rising up to the top, for example, is normally a sign of liver dysfunction. Until you tackle the root cause of the problem, the headaches will continue.

I'm not advocating that you go around in continual pain, but people have medicated themselves so much that they no longer have any connection with the pain they are feeling. Analgesics just raise the threshold of your pain levels, so you have to feel more severe pain in order to be aware of it. Headaches and migraines have different sources and causes. Hormones, stress, food, alcohol, tiredness, allergies or a combination of any of these factors can be responsible.

Apart from taking painkillers, most people deal with a headache by feeding it, saying that having an empty stomach is the reason for their pain. Actually, we usually get head pain if we are dehydrated, not when we need food. The next time you are suffering from this malaise, or you feel a migraine coming on, make sure you have drunk enough water, think about what and how much you've eaten in the preceding four or so days, and how your bowels have performed or not. Elimination is a key factor, and for many this is a major reason for all sorts of so-called mystery complaints. Add fatigue, pressure and stress, and you have the perfect ingredients for headaches, stomach aches, nausea and diarrhoea. People who take laxatives regularly create dehydration and nutrient deficiency as well as weakening the colon's natural mechanisms, so are also likely to be sufferers.

If any of this applies to you, you need to drink plenty of water, with a small teaspoon of cider vinegar added on occasion, and sip slowly, half an hour after a meal, to neutralize any acids and aid digestion. Also take homeopathic remedies that have been specifically prescribed for you, and let your system filter the water through before you eat.

My stomach, to the left of my solar plexus, directly under the rib cage, usually lets me know when my digestive system gets stuck. If I press certain spots, hold the pressure there and take a deep breath in, then slowly let the breath out and press a little bit harder, that area usually starts to gurgle and release.

Get to know where your triggers are, so you can help your body release rubbish. For extra help, support and personal knowledge, use cranial osteopathy, acupuncture and deep tissue massage, as all of these are very effective on a sluggish lymph, and specific organs, meridians and muscles that are blocked. Chinese herbal concoctions from a reputable source can also be extremely helpful.

There are, however, a number of people who do a version of all this already, but still suffer. If that is so, here are some other potential causes of pain that may be worth checking out:
• Mercury toxicity (from amalgams or vaccinations).
• Other metal and liquid pollutant poisoning. This may affect people who work in factories with solvents and/or petrochemicals, or who are exposed to radiation in airports.
• Any bad falls, knocks from animals, operations, dental work or car accidents.
• Hormonal imbalances when women experience pain at exactly the same time every month, in line with their menstrual cycle.
• Dentistry where teeth have been extracted, or orthodontic work where your bite has been distorted, causing tension to certain areas of the skull.
• The last, and sometimes most puzzling reason, is any trauma, physical or emotional, which you won't necessarily know or be aware of. If you suspect this might be the case, then BEST (see page 36) and ART (see page 66) should together, or separately, sort out the problem.

All of the above can be checked by ART and other tests recommended in Chapter 3.

Minimizing Pain
Whatever the root cause, you must take the utmost care with your food, hydration, consumption of alcohol and sugar, plus your elimination process, sleep and stress. A combination of stretching and weight training, using your chosen breathing technique, will also improve your general circulation, with the added benefit of increasing your oxygen intake. This is a great way to reduce pain levels.

Home Environment

This is one area of life that, if not organized, clean, tidy and well-equipped, will let everything else down. Along with emotional challenges, I would say that a disorganized home environment is the main reason why people don't stick to a course of action, remain stressed and never seem to get on top of anything, especially losing weight.

There is nothing better than having a thorough clear out and clean, followed by a re-organization and a few house rules. (Blimey, I sound like my mother!) Seriously though, the state that some people live in, in this day and age, can be quite shocking.

Even if you don't have lots of money, your standards don't have to drop. It doesn't cost much to give the place a lick of fresh paint and it costs nothing to do a really good purge. Whether you are a student, young single adult, married with children or a senior person, if you follow the steps below not only will your home be better organized, but you are likely to feel more mentally organized as you have created physical and mental space in your everyday life.

To begin:
• Make a list of everything that needs your attention – include cleaning, tidying and general organization.
• Go through your wardrobe and divide your clothes into sections – dresses, trousers, shirts, coats, jackets, suits, outfits, sweaters, t-shirts, gym wear, shoes, boots and accessories.
• Take a careful look at each section and decide what you want to give away, sell, throw out or donate to a charity shop; need to wash or have dry-cleaned; or need to mend.
• Put all the clothes you aren't keeping or that need attention into separate bin liners, and put the filled bags straight into the car or out of the way.
• Clean your cupboards with disinfectant and dry them, then put everything you are keeping back in its proper section. Shoe boxes make an ideal container for underwear, socks and tights and help to maintain order.
• Next, go into the kitchen and throw everything out that is past its use-by date. Be ruthless and get rid of old vitamins, medicines and foodstuffs that are anything other than good and nutritious.
• Do the same in the bathroom cabinet, dressing room and living room, sorting bookshelves and drawers and clearing out old magazines, broken objects and discarded presents – general clutter that has built up on your display units.
• Once this is done organize your stationery, address books and diary (buying new ones if necessary) and get up to date with all your paperwork and bills.
• Finally, clean and re-arrange each room to your liking, if necessary buying new sheets and towels and kitchen utensils.
• Remember, be ruthlessly unsentimental. Take anything you don't like or know that you're never going to use to a charity shop.

Once organized, it's then just a matter of maintenance. Plus you're far more likely to feel naturally motivated to move on to the next steps in taking care of yourself.

Bathing

Have you ever stopped to think why, when you have a quick shower or bath at the end of your day, no matter how exhausted you feel, it really helps to perk you up? This is partly because you have got rid of the grime, pollution and your own toxic sweat, but also because your muscles let go of the day's built-up tension.

Your skin is your largest organ and its primary purpose is to excrete toxins. No matter whether you lie in bed all day or are rushing round, your body will be emitting toxins. The chemical build-up in all of our systems, coupled with whatever is going on with our hormones, plus our nutrition, alcohol intake and, for some, tobacco, all make for quite a heavy cocktail. Learning to get rid of that each day, by washing and scrubbing properly, has its merits.

The difference a really good bath makes to the quality of your sleep and to recuperation, helping to stave of infections and colds by releasing muscle tension and fatigue and increasing circulation, is immense.

Showers are great for the morning, and are better than nothing if you don't have a bath. If I only have access to a shower, I usually sit on the floor anyway. Another idea is to attach a wooden shelf at seat height to perch on in the shower.

Bathing is where you learn how to pick yourself up when your energy is flagging, or when you are going through a really hard time emotionally. It is also an extremely important part of successfully getting through illness and recuperation.

Skin Brushing

Skin brushing isn't just for clearing cellulite, it's also a great way to get the circulation going, encouraging any rubbish that's trapped within the layers of the skin to come to the surface and clearing any little pimply areas on the backs of legs, arms and the bottom. Men are always surprised how good they feel after doing this, and comment particularly on the increase in energy that skin brushing results in. For many women who have recently given birth this can be useful towards getting the feeling back in their pelvic floor. Brushing, which should be done on dry skin before exfoliating, can at first be carried out daily and then anywhere between one to four times a week.

Brushing upwards, start on the fingers and hands, then up the arms on to the shoulders and neck, taking care to brush each area thoroughly. Don't rush or be overly aggressive, it will take a week to get used to the abrasiveness; your skin should just feel tingly.

Then start on your feet and ankles, going up the calves, on to the thighs, round to the buttocks (using circular movements), then on to the base of the spine, brushing upwards. Stomachs are optional and should be left to last.

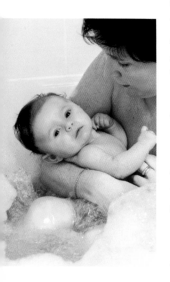

New mother Ghislaine and her newborn baby, Scarlet, relaxing in a hydrotherapy bath. We used a combination of specially formulated natural baby oils and the hydrotherapy to encourage Scarlet to sleep. She fell asleep immediately afterwards, which was a miracle as Scarlet usually fights sleep both during the day and the night.

Next you should exfoliate fully on dry or damp skin. One of my favourite ranges for this is the Calming, Clearing or Warming Organic Body Polishes made by Trillium Herbal Company and Bharti Vyas. I also like Vyas's new body skin polisher. (See Chapter 7 for recommended products.)

Bath Routine

When it comes to daily bathing, put something lovely in the bath, even if you are just in and out in 10 minutes. Use a loofah and body shampoo rigorously all over and rinse off thoroughly. Ren have an excellent choice of body shampoo and Louise Galvin has just brought out a combined hand and body wash to go with her chemical-free shampoo, conditioner and hair mask. If you apply lotion afterwards, this will be more than enough for maintenance.

For a once-a-week or every two-week pamper, follow the routine given below. At the same time, you can if you want apply a mask, either while in the bath or afterwards relaxing on the bed.

For a relaxing bath either use the following on their own or mix a couple together: Moor mud; Tidman's Sea Salt; Alkabath Alkaline bath salts by Organ; the Organic Pharmacy's Organic Rosemary, Lemon Grass, Pine and Eucalyptus bath salts; Himalayan Crystal Bath Salts; organic lemon juice. (Lemons are great for extra cleansing under the arms, and for rubbing on spots if they have a head and need drawing to the surface; toothpaste is also good for this.)

If I want to add something to open up the airways, relax my muscles or stimulate my system, I will use any of the bath products by Nectarome. Their body massage oils are superb as well.

Ideally you should stay in the bath for 20–50 minutes. Have a bottle of water handy, perhaps with some added selectrolytes, Antitox drops by Futureplex or similar drops by the Organic Pharmacy. As soon as you begin to feel overheated, it is important that you put in as much cold water as you need to be wholly comfortable, also allowing any minerals from your chosen products to be absorbed through the skin by osmosis.

When you have finished wallowing, use either a natural loofah or a slightly abrasive sponge and a body shampoo to scrub yourself with.

When you've dried yourself off, apply a body lotion or oil. If you want something rich that smells delightful, the Green People have two wonderful ointment-type body oils, one soothing and the other stimulating.

When you are feeling unwell, pamper yourself as above but leave out the face mask and exfoliation. Do soak in the salts or mud and also dose yourself up with Bioforce C&F Complex as directed on the packaging. If you feel you are coming down with a cold, flu or sore throat, gargling with Himalayan salt or any other pure salts dissolved in water and getting an early night should help you feel better. Continue pampering for three to five days if you are really on the edge. For nasty headaches, stomach upsets or injuries, use specifically prescribed homeopathic remedies. Salts and mud are fantastic if you have back pain or other injuries.

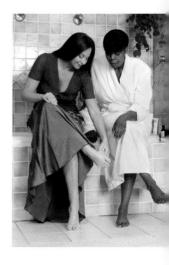

Thirty-five-year-old Jocelyn works hard and plays hard. Carole is showing Jocelyn how to pamper herself. We are getting used to the idea of being pampered, but we still don't take enough care of ourselves on a daily basis.

The most important thing to remember is that when your system is crashing, with colds, flu, stomach bugs and constant minor illnesses, you have to go to bed. There is nothing like sleep, lots of water, natural remedies, baths and relaxation in front of the television or with a book to get you back on the road to feeling really well – and probably better than you have felt in a long time. We put far too much emphasis on keeping everything together and often boasting that we never get ill... Allowing your system to break down and for you to recognize its needs is the best way of building your immune system and ensuring that you feel healthy again.

Massage

Massage is an extremely effective way to aid detoxification, relaxation and help the body recover from injury and day-to-day wear and tear.

One of the most important points is to be comfortable with whoever is treating you. In an ideal world, therapists would not smoke or take drugs and their alcohol consumption would be minimal so that no rubbish is transferred to the recipient's body. The therapist also benefits from this, as body work is very labour-intensive.

For therapists who also personally train their clients, massage gives them a reference point as to how the body they are treating is functioning in all areas of elimination, digestion and fluid retention, where tension is held and how that affects the client's breathing and posture, which side they favour, and more.

Depending on the type of massage chosen you can achieve three things at once: drainage and stimulation of the lymphatic and digestive systems; alleviation of tension in all muscle groups, resulting in a change in the structure of the muscle; and, just as importantly, relaxation. But a practitioner with these combined skills can be hard to find. Masseurs' initial training on anatomy and contraindications is thorough and consistent. However, in terms of application and manipulation, initial know-how and skill can be patchy. Most trainees aren't taught how to use their body weight effectively for their own posture or the pressure they put on the body they are treating, nor are they shown how to distribute the strength used between fingers, hands and torso. Being able to achieve depth and strength when working on a person's body does not rely on the masseur being bulky, strong or tall, but rather on the position they stand or sit in when massaging. It is also important for them to position themselves correctly so they can apply pressure without bruising their client.

No matter how much you think you prefer a gentle, stroking massage, it really doesn't bring the same benefits that you can derive from a firm or deep massage. The exceptions to this are pressure-point treatments such as acupressure or shiatsu. For pain relief or any improvement in your body's filtration and muscular systems, where massage is concerned, there must be a certain degree of depth.

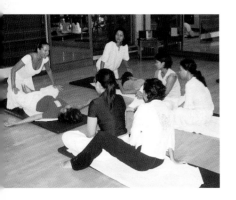

Carole is working with a group of therapists from all over eastern Asia, concentrating on the differences in stretching and manipulating Western as opposed to Eastern bodies. She dedicates part of the session to giving advice about their own nutrition, posture, breathing and energy levels, to ensure that each of these therapists understands the importance of looking after themselves.

Ideally, a massage should never be limited by time. To get the most out of it, you should either have a bath, steam, or at the very least a shower immediately prior to the massage. When being massaged every part of the body should be included, especially the extremities. Reiki is a great way to finish a massage, leaving recipients with a deep sense of relaxation, which they are left to come out of in their own time.

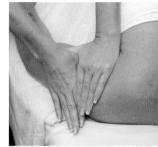

Recipients of massage often comment that no other part of the body seems to be worked on as thoroughly as the back and shoulders. Yet massaging the feet, which have pressure points corresponding to all parts of the body, and the legs, which carry your whole weight and are responsible for at least a third of the drainage of your lymphatic system, is of the outmost importance. That's why I recommend therapists start with the feet and then fully drain the legs. By the time they reach the back, it's much better primed for them to manipulate.

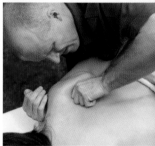

Finding a therapist to work on you the way you would like is usually much easier when you are at home than when you are on holiday. Hotels providing massage and/or spa facilities are often under pressure to ensure they make good profits so their goals may be based on turnover and selling products.

Masseurs have to work in a multifaceted way, hour in, hour out. They are often exhausted, not fed well and have nowhere they can go to recuperate and sleep to replenish their energy. They are allowed on average 50 minutes to do a massage with 10 minutes to get the room ready for the next person. If you're lucky the newest spas may offer you anything up to 75 minutes. Although it is changing, there is a real lack of integration of knowledge and training, and the masseur's own level of health, well-being and fitness isn't taken into account.

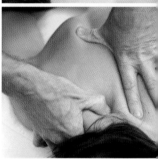

When having a massage don't be afraid to state what you do and don't want done, or stop the massage if it is irritating you. If you aren't sure what products are going to be used on you, take natural organic oils with you. If your health is below par you don't want to use too many essential oils as they will compete with your detoxification process. Neither do you want lots of chemicals or any other noxious substances included in any of your wraps or treatments. This defeats the object of these treatments, and you wouldn't believe the amount of rubbish in most product lines, no matter how natural they are purported to be. (See Chapter 7 for products to take with you.) The spa at Pennyhill Park Hotel, Surrey, is one of the first places to have a range of products that are totally chemical-free. They are designed by Circaroma and will really set a standard for the future of spas in Britain.

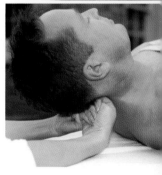

David Brown and Carole using deep tissue technique to stretch out and realign the fibres of the muscles. David works with dancers, singers and athletes to help them recover from injury, and reach their full potential.

When choosing a facial, whatever the product and method, make sure it includes a full lymphatic massage from the chest and top of the arms into the shoulders and neck, then lastly a very thorough drainage of the face. Fifteen minutes is the minimum for this to be fully effective. Products can greatly improve the effects of a facial, but check all the ingredients of the spa's chosen products (usually noxious) and if you aren't happy with their selection take your own masks, exfoliators and oils (see Chapter 7 for suggestions).

Thai Massage

Thai massage incorporates assisted stretching with fast movement manipulation and pummelling. For those who don't like taking their clothes off this form of massage is ideal, as you get to keep them on! The mixture of stretching and manipulation is incredibly beneficial for a tired or under-utilized body, and this is the one massage that usually lasts a decent amount of time.

Anywhere you go in the world and have treatments, I advise that you speak with the manager of the spa upon arrival, or prior to your session, to explain your needs and preferences.

Reflexology

If you are lucky, you can actually combine reflexology with a full body massage. However, reflexology is a complete treatment in itself. It is recommended for all sorts of ailments and by many oncologists for patients undergoing chemotherapy and radiation.

For women during pregnancy and in helping to keep contractions up during labour, reflexology is a very subtle and effective way of diagnosing and treating the body's ailments. Once again though, it's all down to the skill of the practitioner.

Back Care

I still marvel at the number of people who, when they have a back problem, ache or pain in a muscular part of their body, deal with it by going to a doctor and getting painkillers, steroids, injections or resort to surgery without checking out all the options. Before you take any of these actions, I strongly recommend that you fully explore the many other possibilities that have proven with millions of people to be fully effective.

Some back problems can be dealt with relatively quickly while others can go on mysteriously for years even after supposedly trying all available treatments. Many back problems are caused by muscles in the lower lumbar region being too strong, pulling the vertebrae towards each other while the stomach muscles remain weak. This process pinches the nerves, leading to a niggly, achy feeling as the circulation is cut off. The main release for most back troubles is to allow the legs and hip joints to carry the weight of gravity into the ground and in so doing the muscles and vertebrae can be released. It's often the misalignment of the bones that causes the problems as the muscles try to support the body rather than just moving the bones, which is what their job is.

A collapsed pelvic floor, favouring one side of the body more than the other, or the clenching of the gluteus in the buttocks – which 95 per cent of us do, and which shortens the quadriceps significantly – are just a few of the many contributing factors to back problems.

What's happening in your life emotionally may be another factor. Heavy medication, such as continual use of antidepressants, steroids, epidurals and the

• More than 17 million people in the UK suffer from back pain – around 25 per cent of the population – ranking it second only to headaches as the most common site of pain.

like can also be the cause of – or major irritant of – back pain. The cause and severity of a back problem are essential to diagnose before you throw yourself into any set of exercises. In an ideal world disc problems and serious structural injuries to any part of the body would be worked on by a team of professionals including an osteopath, a back exercise specialist and if necessary a surgeon. See www.lonclin.co.uk to find out about the London Spine Clinic.

Posture, breathing and stretching in an asymmetric position (in other words not twisting the pelvis and small of the back out of alignment and learning to isolate the hip flexors) are vital before you try any hyperextension or lifting movements. This process can take anything from two weeks to several months. The muscle fibres in many areas of the body have to increase in mobility and in equality on both sides of the body to safely service strength and cardiovascular activity.

Cranial osteopathy, acupuncture and cognitive kinesiology are just some of the treatments that are incredibly successful at either supporting or rectifying many back problems.

Be aware with any physiotherapy, cranial or osteopathic work that, unless fully explained and justified, you should not have the treatment more than once in a seven-day period. The body needs time to digest a treatment and to rest. Like any form of exercise, the results manifest between sessions.

Increasingly, there are a number of sufferers who have derived no definitive conclusion or sustained results from any of the more physically based treatments, but have found effective relief from BEST and ART, both of which can check and remove any emotional memory causes.

Remember that food can be an irritant to the back. When in pain, do not have any liquids or foods that overheat the blood and cause the muscles to contract, for example sugar, caffeine, alcohol and strong spicy or peppery food – keep it simple.

Also consider changing your chair at work. Many furniture shops supply Balans chairs, amongst other choices, which after the initial adjustment period of three to five days are a godsend. This type of chair angles your back in such a way that your posture can never collapse. Alternatively, use an exercise ball, which is available from most sports and department stores to achieve the same effect. Check also that your bed or mattress are not aggravating the problem.

Finally, whatever treatment or specific problem you have, homeopathy is a very effective support to the whole healing process of the tissues, ligaments and muscles.

Osteopathy And Cranial-sacral Therapy

Even people who know who and where to go when the structural body needs help often wait until the offending problem is extremely bad. Ideally, like a dentist, you should see an osteopath two or three times a year for a thorough check-up – aside from the times when you have a specific problem.

As well as treating back problems and injuries, osteopathy and cranial therapy can also release shortness in the muscles from bad posture. Release work needed in other areas of the body, such as the pelvic floor, stomach, solar plexus, face, skull and any of the joints may effectively alleviate any system in your body that is blocked, which you may have been unaware of. Many years ago, I was very nervous and stressed and my menstrual cycle was late and causing me great discomfort. I went to have a special treatment outside of my normal appointments, and within 24 hours had the result I wanted.

When you have an injury, whether long-standing or immediate, the cause is often not at the site where you actually feel the pain. There are also reverberations that will affect the rest of your body, usually causing your posture to go out of alignment. It's both useful and important to know how to fix and deal with this as well as being made aware of where and what has been affected. The cranial part of an osteopathic treatment prepares the site in case anything more aggressive is needed as well as dealing with the aftershock. Cranial-sacral therapy is commonly used on newborn babies and mothers and is very beneficial after going to the dentist/hygienist and after any operative procedures to realign the cranium and structural body.

Immediately after your treatment and for the next 24 hours, watch your intake of food and drink as you don't want your system to have to fight against alcohol, caffeine and rich, fatty foods. Drink plenty of water and do not do any physical exercise after the treatment on that day. Ideally, at the end of the day you should go home, take a bath and relax.

Between The Sheets

People boast about how little sleep they need or can get by on, as if it's something to be proud of. Yet sleep is when the body does most of its repair work and in this day and age, people need more sleep than ever before. Sleep is when you emotionally discharge and download your feelings. If you have teenagers who sleep until noon on weekends, don't berate them but check whether they need time away from their mobile phone, computer or peers in order to recharge their batteries.

Many studies over the years have confirmed that few people are free of sleep problems. When tired or distressed, people can toss and turn 140–160 times a night, which in itself is stressful. More than half of all car accidents are caused by tiredness or drowsiness. Fatigue leaves people unable to function properly at work, unable to focus or concentrate, and most of all unable to heal properly or recharge their batteries. When sleep-deprived, we become irritable, bad tempered and generally difficult to be around.

A bad night's sleep also distorts your viewpoint, makes you feel more emotionally vulnerable and is one of our nation's biggest problems. Why don't people sleep well?

There's a variety of reasons including discomfort from pain in the body, stress from work or family, empathic or electromagnetic stress. For example two of the worst things you can have in your bedroom are an electric blanket or a water bed.

But why, I hear you cry, when they are so wonderful to sleep on? Consider this. When you lie down in bed, your body wishes to relax into a calming arcadian brain rhythm of about seven cycles per second. Your electric blanket and waterbed are plugged into the wall and have electrical circuits running through them at a frequency of between 56 and 60 cycles per second. So the body is immediately put under a huge amount of stress, you cannot relax properly and therefore are unable to get the quality of sleep you need. If the cells in your body become swollen due to stress, they will be painful because they lack oxygen and are acidic, which in turn creates general discomfort and an inability to lie still.

To sleep well we also need to make sure that we have emptied our mental dustbins at the end of the day so that we can avoid over-stimulation of all our systems. Often you read that watching television before going to bed can erode a good night's sleep, but that reading can make you sleepy. The fact is both can have either effect, it all depends on you. Eating too late and drinking alcohol, sugar and caffeine at night are all factors that can make the difference between getting a good night's sleep or not. If you sleep all the way through the night but wake up feeling less than refreshed that is not considered to be a good night's sleep.

Oxygen supply and the pineal gland, which is in charge of all healing and energy systems, are key elements that often get missed when trying to sort out what's going wrong. The brain and body need the right amount of oxygen stimulation to be able to fall asleep. Hence another reason why exercise at the right time of the day for your body is so important.

The reason I advise people to bathe before they go to sleep, no matter how late, even if it's just for five minutes, is that it's good to take the weight off your feet and hot water cleanses and relaxes the muscles. Your breathing changes and your body is prepared to get the most out of the night's rest.

If you have a working lifestyle that demands long hours and heavy input, then sleep has to be your priority. Socializing too much during the week will mean that you are always running on empty, having to rely on your adrenal glands which in turn affects your immune system and creates cravings for coffee and sugar to keep you going, which eventually causes your system to crash. This is a horrible way to feel and live from day to day.

So if your body is saying: 'Lie down, I need to sleep' – listen to it. It is not a sin to have an early night more than once in a while, in fact whatever is needed to service your daily output.

When you go to sleep, the circadian rhythm of your brain – the natural rate at which you function – should calm down to a gentle undulation. In a properly deep state of sleep the pineal gland is activated. If this doesn't happen then you will wake up in the morning feeling dreadful, your batteries will not have been recharged and nothing in your body will have had a chance to heal.

Sleep is a wonderful restorer of biological energy. Too little and your immune system is compromised and you become weak. You will be unable to efficiently eliminate toxins from the body, will be invaded by micro-organisms and will be more prone to the degenerative disorders that prevail with the onset of old age. It is the sleep period that also controls and promotes the release of melatonin and growth hormones.

Melatonin is known to have anti-cancer properties and to help control endocrine function. It also has anti-ageing properties, assists immune function and helps control respiration. In order to promote melatonin, you need to sleep in complete darkness.

In fact, where you sleep and how you sleep is incredibly important in general. One of the best ways to naturally assist this process is to sleep on a magnetic mattress pad, widely used in insomniac clinics in the US. The north side of a magnet helps to neutralize body acidity, which is great for people under enormous stress or who are acidic through degenerative disorders such as arthritis.

Magnets also help to relax the organs, tissues and muscles so that the body can get to sleep more quickly and deeply. If used in conjunction with a magnetic pillow pad, the north-facing magnets can assist in lowering the circadian rhythm of the brain so you switch off more effectively. This is a much more natural way to assist in sleeping than using sleeping pills. Magnetic mattresses and pillows boost the immune system, help to rebalance hormones and have many other benefits. If you wish to purchase one then ensure that you find a supplier who is an accredited magnet therapist. A good product should have magnets of at least 3,900 gauss in strength – if it is less it will not have the same benefit. There are a few contraindications too, such as having a pacemaker or being pregnant, so check with your supplier.

Settling Into A Routine

Simona Arneodo is one of the world's top maternity consultants. Coming from a typical Italian family-orientated background, she has always been fascinated by children (and babies in particular), and the various strands of thought concerning their upbringing during the early developmental stages.

Since 1992, Simona has worked as a full-time private maternity nurse and consultant, based in London but travelling all over the world, helping parents with the care and development of their newborn babies. She specializes in sleep and feed training, weaning and diet. Simona says: 'I have researched countless theories and studies concerning childcare, and although the majority provide some very sound advice, such information is often conflicting and I can understand why parents become a little confused. Throughout my years working with babies and parents, I have formulated my own ideas and have successfully developed a method and approach that produces truly rewarding results. Although I firmly believe that babies greatly benefit from a well-structured routine, I also believe that parents are ultimately the ones who should decide which path to follow, and my methods always provide a degree of flexibility to accommodate and assist their wishes.

'A common myth about routines is that they prevent parents from attending to the baby's needs, which may seem a little harsh. In fact, though, a properly constructed routine merely sets regular periods of time for sleep and for stimulating, relaxing and nurturing your baby. Babies love to know what's coming next. A stable routine reassures them and helps them to become independent, confident and relaxed, which ultimately has a positive effect on their personality.

'Many baby care books claim it is impossible or unwise to put a newborn baby into a routine during the first few weeks, and that by doing so you could cause psychological damage. Such claims have not been proven, and in many years of personal experience I have found this is simply not the case. In fact, I have discovered that babies who have been put into a sympathetic routine by structuring the right feeding and sleeping patterns from the start develop into well-adjusted, happy children.

'You also constantly hear from many well-intentioned advisors that unpredictable, inconsistent early feeding and sleeping patterns are normal and that things will naturally get better and in time your baby will become settled. The truth though is by neglecting this issue in the early days, many bad habits may develop; if your baby has not been guided in the right way, this may cause further complications by creating long-term sleeping and feeding problems.

'One of the greatest gifts you can give your baby is to teach him to fall asleep by himself — to be a "self-soother". Babies are creatures of habit, learning by example and association, and establishing the right sleeping associations from the very start encourages your baby to become a self-soother.

'The benefits for the parents of a routine are also tremendous; the usual stress and turmoil associated with a new baby is greatly reduced, bringing harmony and confidence to the home. Parents become positive and feel in control and relaxed, creating a comfortable reassuring atmosphere, which is passed on to the baby. It's not simply a case of ignoring your baby and allowing him to scream and cry until he is exhausted, but establishing proper sleep and feeding patterns and developing a routine to suit your baby. Your baby should not be compared to others; each baby is an individual and will respond in different ways.'

Simona's main tips are: Food does not equal love. An unsettled baby is not always a hungry baby. Establishing a routine will teach you to recognize your baby's different types of crying and attend to his needs with confidence. Babies love to know what's coming next. It reassures them and helps them to become independent, confident and relaxed, which ultimately has a positive effect on their personality. Don't compare your baby to others — babies are individuals and will respond in different ways. Pick your own path and learn to trust your own judgment. You will make mistakes, but fortunately babies are very adaptable and resilient and will quickly and happily adjust. By following a routine you'll soon realize you still have a life. Feeding your baby is an important connection and should be unhurried and quiet — a perfect moment to share and get to know

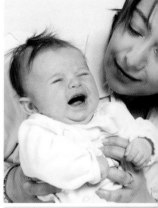

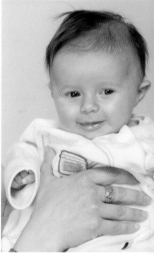

Simona Arneodo is one of the world's top maternity nurses who specializes in sleep and feeding, weaning and nutrition.

each other Avoid rocking, feeding and dummies to get your baby to sleep. A massage after a bath is a perfect way to relax your baby and to promote and enhance a bonding relationship. Don't over-stimulate your baby or let him become overtired, he will be impossible to settle. All babies have bad days as well as good days, but always think of tomorrow as a good day. Value your baby's need for independence. Even babies need their own space, so allow them to explore this new world by themselves from time to time. Don't neglect yourself or your partner – although you have become a mother, don't stop being a wife or companion.

If you follow these rules from the start, later you'll be able to break some, and still have a happy, well-adjusted child.

Travel And Jet Lag

Have you ever wondered why travelling takes so much out of you? Apart from the mad rush to get everything completed at home and work, packing and so on, there is a whole other factor that bombards and traumatizes the body. When you walk into an airport and on to a plane, you are surrounded by electromagnetic fields and radiation which come off all the display boards, communication systems, security check-ins and X-ray machines. Then, when you are on the plane, you're scrunched up in the seat, the air is stagnant and you've got the food to contend with. So when your skin seems to age like the aliens in *Star Trek*, your bowels play havoc and your water retention seems worse than ever, this will give you a clue as to why.

Still, the excitement and adventure far outweigh the cons. All we have to do is be aware and be prepared. So what can you do? For three days before flying, take antioxidant supplements, if you are not already doing so. For anyone who suffers from back pain or backache, take the recommended dosage of arnica 6 or 6x on the day of travel and the day after. Silver colloidal, which is a liquid form of a highly concentrated, 98 per cent absorbable mineral supplement, is another travel gem. Take it prior to travelling and throughout the holiday too. On the day of travel and the next day take the recommended dose of Bush Flower Travel Essence mixed with the correct amount of selectrolytes and water.

Because of what you are being exposed to and the trauma of travelling, the lack of oxygen and dehydration, your acidity levels need to be lowered. Taking chlorella will not only help to keep your alkaline status in check but is very effective should you pick up any parasites along the way.

Wear natural fibres when travelling because material such as nylon is suffocating and you need as much oxygen as you can get. Unfortunately, nylon does not mix well with our natural pH and tends to end up being rather smelly.

I also advise caution where aircraft food is concerned. You have already been in contact with radiation – do you really want to eat it as well? Take a light and healthy snack on your flight – one that will satisfy you and digest easily. And if you want to feel as good as possible, don't even think about drinking caffeine or alcohol. You may not realize it, but you will not be pleasant to sit next to.

The toiletries that are so kindly provided to you by some airlines, including the face and hand wipes, are really cheap, but they are full of rubbish and you don't need to use them. Take your own supplies from our recommended list in Chapter 7. In short, resist the temptation to stuff everything into your mouth and keep every freebie. It's simply not worth it. (I guess I've now blown my chances of being upgraded!)

Taking Care In The Sun

The last 18 months in particular have seen the great sun debate fire in many different directions. To sunblock or not sunblock, that is the question? Should you go in the sun or should you not? It is true that our ozone layer and the dangers of the sun are very real. However, it is also the case that unwanted conditions such as rickets and depression are caused by low or no exposure to sunlight. Too many people who do go in the sun are in poor condition and don't prepare themselves properly. I believe that this has a major effect on the outcome of how a person reacts to the sun.

Dosing ourselves up on alcohol, fizzy drinks, fried and rich food, plus ice creams and ice-cold drinks while on holiday create a perfect opportunity for our systems to react as soon as the heat of the sun hits us, let alone any of the rays. Think of it like a steamroom or sauna – instant detoxification plus dehydration if you're not a water drinker.

Add to which we then douse ourselves in sun creams full of petrochemicals and a whole host of other ingredients and it is no wonder that reams of people are paranoid. The opportunities that holidays can provide for regeneration are many, but there are some rules that you have to adhere to. Your intake of water has to be good all year round, and particularly when you are in the sun. Also take some selectrolytes if you dehydrate or suffer from headaches or dizziness.

If you allow yourself to eat healthily, drink lots of water, relax and sleep in the shade or in the sun during the safe part of the day when the rays are milder and you are more used to it, deep tiredness as well as water retention and excess weight can fall away. You can still derive nutrient benefits from the sun as long as you don't overdo it.

A few weeks before your holiday start to cut out the substances your body doesn't need, get some decent R and R, start skin brushing and exfoliating your body and face regularly, and once your skin has got used to the sun continue to exfoliate on holiday. All this will ensure an even tan and guard against peeling and patchiness.

Use one of the recommended brands of body oil or lotion (see Chapter 7) and make sure you use it after bathing or showering. Steam and sauna treatments help greatly in getting your body ready for coping with the detox effect that happens in a hot climate, as does taking a good-quality antioxidant. Organic Pharmacy does an excellent one.

As well as taking a good antioxidant and an essential fatty acid supplement, there is a supplement called Source of Life made by Nature Plus that you should take a month before going away. Children should take BioCare's Vitasorb Multi before and during the break. Also take Sol 30, a homeopathic remedy, twice weekly during the lead up to your holiday and daily on holiday.

Preparing your body in this way, before going on holiday, will make a significant difference to your health while you are away. I know that there are many attractive-looking products in chemists and department stores (as well as a lot of cheap and nasty ones), but I really would advise that you are not seduced into buying any of these. If you want a product that will get your skin ready for the sun use Sun Love by Energys, which prepares the skin by supplying it with extra melanin, the body's own tanning agent. Argon oil, aloe vera and vitamins A and E are all included in this product. Just as importantly it contains no titanium dioxide, one of the numbers of chemicals found in many sun screens that are now suspected of being carcinogenic.

If you really want to use fake tan, use Lavera's, who also do natural sun products.

Of course, it really is essential to know when to get out of the sun and to build your exposure to it slowly. If necessary break up the holiday by having the odd day where you stay mainly in the shade. Your body will respond to this a lot better than if you suffocate yourself for long hours in the sun using a heavy chemicalized sunblock. You can't use a cream or take a pill to stop dehydration, sun stroke, burning and more serious knock-on effects.

First Aid

Each of us would benefit hugely by having the skills that can make the difference between life and death – knowing the basics to aid people after car accidents, heart attacks, strokes, epileptic fits, alcohol poisoning, asthma attacks, fights and, in this day and age, even bombs and terror attacks. Being able to keep someone alive until they reach a hospital, or an ambulance arrives, is quite an awesome feat.

Yet First Aid has had a consistently poor image over the last 50 years, and is often considered to be of little value as a skill – until it is suddenly and urgently needed. Until comparatively recently, it was seen primarily as being about tea and sympathy. Yet First Aid is in fact a branch of medicine.

The simple definition of First Aid is 'knowing what to do, and being able to do it when an accident or sudden illness occurs, using the facilities and materials that are available at the time'. Equally important is knowing what should *not* be done, so that further damage is not caused.

Some of the most common First Aid myths include:
• Tipping a person's head back in cases of nosebleeds – this may choke them.
• Putting creams or lotions on burns – there is nothing more likely to become infected than a burn, and whatever is put on will have to be taken off when the patient reaches hospital.

Bullet wound to the shoulder.

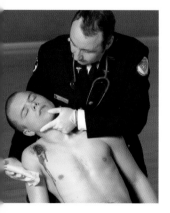

• Putting spoons and other objects into the mouth of someone suffering an epileptic fit to prevent them from swallowing or biting their tongue. In reality, you will either choke them or break their teeth. The tongue is attached to the lower jaw, so it is almost impossible to swallow it.

• Giving cups of tea, water or brandy to someone who has had an accident and is in shock. Even in mild shock, the digestive system shuts down, and anything eaten or drunk is likely to be regurgitated. When the injury is severe enough to require surgery, stomach content and anaesthetic are generally incompatible, so giving drinks can delay surgery.

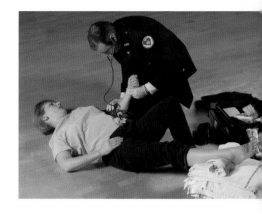

Foot or ankle fracture.

First Aid And Touch

My First Aid trainers, Donald and Lesley, told me they never fail to be surprised by how many people are incredibly uncomfortable at being touched or touching others. They find that by the end of a training course, many participants are completely unrecognizable, leaving with a self-esteem and confidence not present when they arrived. They also teach youngsters in remand for committing violent crimes, and find they have a completely new attitude and respect for other people after doing the course. First Aid training gives children and teenagers in general a real advantage in understanding and being comfortable with the issue of physical contact.

Although the definition of First Aid may sound simple and mere common sense, in reality its practice demands knowledge, skill and imagination, as well as the confidence to use it in a medical emergency.

The main aims are to preserve life, prevent a condition from getting worse and promote recovery. First Aid is also not necessarily something we always do on other people. In some cases it will be a case of self-aid, and should therefore be considered as part of our personal survival kit. A First Aid course takes between three and five days – a relatively short time to learn the skills that could save lives. So don't think: 'It's never going to happen to me' – and sign up for a First Aid course.

If you are thinking of doing a training course – which I'd strongly recommend – you should think about whether it would be primarily for work, home or leisure. Any trainers you contact will help you identify the form of training for your particular needs.

If you need the course for work purposes, contact the Health and Safety Executive at Quay House, Quay Street, Manchester, M3 3JB; tel 0161 952 8200 and they will advise you of your local registered First Aid at Work training providers. If your requirements are for home or leisure, then try Yellow Pages or go to www. artcon-heartstart.com.

A Modern Approach To Menopause

The menopause is a natural process of hormonal changes, signifying a time of life when the female body is switching over to a different rhythm. A common question is that, if this is a natural process, why does modern society react and interfere in the way that it does? This would be an entirely valid point if we lived in a more naturally healthy world. As we've already mentioned though, our environment is polluted with chemicals that infiltrate the food chain and upset the body's natural adaptive processes and hormonal function.

Also, we now live to a much older age, and the longer we live without glandular hormonal support and balance, the more our bodily functions gradually deteriorate. This is a very slow and subtle process, usually manifesting 10–15 years after the onset of menopause.

Yet most women in today's world have no intention of gradually fading away when they reach their fifities or sixties. On the contrary, many want to take on ambitious projects with all the stresses that can go with it. They expect their mental faculties and body to perform just as they did when they were in their thirties.

The design of the body is very fine and delicate in its mechanism for hormonal balance, and is not easy to mimic. For this reason, it's best to help the body up to 10 years before the menopause, maintaining its ability for balance by taking good care of it in all respects.

This involves looking after what and how we eat, doing weight-bearing exercise, removing or minimizing any toxic load including mercury amalgam fillings, supporting the adrenal gland, stabilizing blood sugar levels to avoid the stress of hypoglycaemia, and drainage remedies to maximize toxin elimination, even on a cellular level.

Chinese and Japanese women have a good approach to keeping their bodies in balance. Even from a dietary point of view, they naturally do not eat many dairy products, potatoes, bread or pasta. They are culturally more aware of how to support their bodies using herbs and foods as medicine. So, for example, they know what herbs to put in their soups and stews to support what they regard as the kidney 'essence', which is primarily what gets depleted as menopause approaches. The Chinese medical philosophy on the menopause is also amazingly accurate in both describing and treating this process.

Stabilizing blood sugar levels is also an important part of the treatment or management of menopause, particularly in minimizing the frequency or extent of hot flushes.

The HRT Debate

The jury's out on whether it's advisable for women to use hormone replacement therapy (HRT) and if so, for how long. Some fortunate women hardly notice menopause, while others suffer the most appalling symptoms. The worse the symptoms, the more the need to consider HRT. For all the raging controversy, it's still true to say that for those women whose lives are shattered by the mental, emotional and physical effects of menopause, hormone replacement within a limited timeframe can be a life saver. Women who have had a hysterectomy or other similar form of surgical intervention at an early age can also benefit greatly.

At the time of writing, the NHS guidelines are that severe menopausal symptoms can be treated by HRT, provided the patient has been fully informed of the risks involved, particularly the increased risk of cancer.

It's also currently recommended that women should take HRT for no more than five years and, during that time, they should drink as little alcohol as possible. As with the Pill, the oestrogen in HRT is believed to increase the risk of blood clots – or thrombosis.

Each individual woman has to decide for herself what she should do, in consultation with a doctor she trusts. Personal and family medical history is the first guide to whether HRT is an option. Your doctor will want to know if you have any history of heart problems, thrombosis, abnormal blood pressure, arthritis, osteoporosis, depression, mood swings, joint pain, low energy, emotional disturbances or relationship problems – a big spectrum to view.

I strongly recommend carefully exploring all the alternatives. Seek out a good homeopath and nutritionist and see what he/she recommends, and ask your GP about bio-identical, or natural, hormone therapy. Most will not have heard of it, but there are a small number of doctors in the UK who now prescribe these alternatives to synthetic HRT manufactured by pharmaceutical companies.

Natural hormones come in different preparations as pessaries, creams for topical use, tablets, as oil-based capsules or as sublingual drops.

But taking hormones, even natural hormones, is not always a straightforward matter. A key organ for processing hormones adequately is the liver. If it's congested or sluggish then taking hormones is not the priority – treating the liver is. A congested, sluggish liver unfortunately does not show on medical blood tests or scans, but does show clearly when tested energetically such as with electrodermal screening.

The priority always has to be to first ensure adequate flow of blood and the smooth running of all other channels in the body especially the elimination channels, which primarily include the gut and lymphatic system.

Taking HRT should also involve looking at more than just the two female hormones, progesterone and oestrogen. It also needs to include checking and treating deficiencies of thyroid hormones as well as testosterone and other androgens, both of which have important functions, even in a woman, for protecting the bones, heart and breasts.

A useful test for assessing hormone requirements is a urine hormone profile which gives information not just about a panel of up to eight hormones, but also important guidance about the relationship of these hormones to each other. Not only is this test helpful to have as a baseline, it can also show how your hormone prescription needs to be adjusted during the course of taking HRT.

Whatever choices you make, update regularly. Visit your GP to get your hormone levels tested, and check on the health of your breasts, heart and lungs, your bone density levels and your weight.

Remember, too, the benefits of acupuncture, cranial treatment, massage and other hands-on therapies. Also remember to keep updating your knowledge of information on HRT versus alternative support. If you're on HRT, keep asking and checking if and when you can reduce the medication.

Recommended Tests:
• Urine hormone profile to see and treat exactly what shows up as deficient.
• Thyroid function tests.
• Hair mineral analysis to check for presence of toxic metals and mineral status. This test will also give an indication about thyroid and adrenal function.
• Regular bone density scans to screen for osteoporosis.
• Regular thermal imaging scans to detect early abnormalities that may develop in the breasts.
• Regular pelvic scans to check the ovaries and thickness of the lining of the womb as well as for fibroids.

For a premenopausal chart and how to survive the menopause through nutrition see www.lifesmart.co.uk.

A Modern Approach To The Andropause

The process of the male andropause is exactly the same as the menopause, with glandular function slowing down and creating a gradual decline in the level of the male hormones DHEA and testosterone.

Men are affected in a similar way to women, except that it is not so dramatic, with hot flushes, night sweats and disturbed sleep.

Generally, men experience a drop in stamina and energy levels at this time. In the Chinese medical system, it is men's kidney energy that declines during andropause, and they also often accumulate heat in the liver.

While for women, it is the breasts that are most vulnerable to hormonal changes and accumulation of toxins in the body, in men it is the prostate gland. As with women during menopause, the changes to the prostate gland start very gradually and subtly. Symptoms of a weak prostate gland can even be an early signal indicating the onset of andropause.

Urine hormone profile tests on men who are entering or in andropause often show not only low levels of DHEA and testosterone, but also low levels of progesterone and normal to high levels of oestrogen. It is these normal to high levels of oestrogen, combined with low levels of progesterone, that contribute to prostate enlargement. Just as women need a small amount of male hormones to keep the other hormones in balance, so men need a small amount of the female hormones, especially progesterone, to keep their hormone profile in balance.

Apart from being influenced by hormonal changes, the prostate gland is also a common area for the accumulation of metals and fungal growth, both of which can only be detected energetically using electrodermal screening or ART (see page 66). Metal accumulation can be confirmed with a tissue hair mineral analysis, and is often caused by mercury amalgam fillings in the mouth.

Recommended Tests:
• Prostate, thyroid and lipid/cholesterol profile.
• Hair mineral analysis for mineral and toxic metal assessment.
• Urine hormone profile.
• Electrodermal screening to check for energetic imbalances.
• Screening for heart disease with blood pressure monitoring and, for diabetes, platelet aggregation and stress ECG.

Mouthing Off

Have you ever had those recurring nightmares where your teeth fall out? You might think that nowadays this predicament would be non-existent, but, in fact, you'd be surprised how prevalent it still is.

For whatever reason, many people do not go to the dentist or hygienist, nor do they take adequate care of their teeth on a daily basis. But once you start to get problems with your teeth and the rot sets in, it is very, very hard to go back. There are millions of people walking around with teeth missing, dentures or caps that have to be renewed. When a mouth goes wrong it can lead to all sorts of trouble in various parts of the body.

An abscess under a tooth can cause very bad head pain to severe nausea, and if not dealt with immediately can lead to abscesses forming in other parts of the body. The mouth can spread poison and decay faster than any other area.

Daily maintenance of flossing and brushing teeth properly is of key importance. I always thought that I took fairly good care of my teeth, until I met a dentist who said their excellent state was due far more to my diet and daily water intake than to the maintenance of healthy gums. Instead of referring me to a hygienist, though, he showed me how to do the Bass toothbrush technique. Of course I argued that I didn't have the time, but he was insistent. As with adopting any habit, once you get into the swing of it, time ceases to be an issue. Here, courtesy of Dr David Harvey Austin, is the technique – which works!

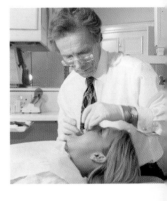

Dr David Harvey Austin checking that a patient has been following his instructions for cleaning their teeth.

Bass Tooth Brushing Technique For Gum Conditioning

Unlike most 'normal' tooth brushing, which only cleans the teeth, this technique is designed to *condition the gum tissues* while *automatically cleaning the teeth*.

When used effectively and regularly, it should prevent the build-up of plaque, which produces inflammation of the gum tissues and a subsequent erosive effect on supporting bone tissue. Long term, this erosion can lead to such a degree of loss that the tooth has to be removed.

Primary Technique

1. Always use a dry toothbrush (no toothpaste) and keep the bristles dry with a tissue.
2. Angle the bristles at 45 degrees down into the gum groove around the teeth and push down very firmly – although it will not happen, imagine you are trying very hard to push the gum further down the teeth (any apparent drop in gum level will only come about as the swollen gum tissues 'shrink' back to normal healthy tissue).
3. While holding the bristles firmly in place, rotate the head of the toothbrush in a circular fashion.
4. Using the coloured middle section of the toothbrush as a guide, move this section from tooth to tooth so that you condition the gum and clean each tooth individually – five circular strokes per tooth (with the overlap that occurs, each tooth will receive 15 strokes in total).
5. Do this in a regular pattern around both the outer and inner surfaces of each tooth and then complete the toothbrushing by giving the biting surfaces a hard 'scrub'.
6. When finished, take a teacup of the hottest water you can bear, add a teaspoon of salt and rinse your mouth thoroughly. This will help with the resolution of both gum soreness and bleeding which you will most probably encounter over the first few days, after which this soreness and bleeding should start to decline.

To be effective, this should be done four times a day for ten days. When the conditioning is complete, maintain gum health by using the secondary technique (opposite) morning and evening (after food).

Accessories to the Gum Conditioning Technique

Disclosing Tablets

1. The sole purpose of these tablets is to let you see *exactly* where the plaque is on your teeth.
2. Crush the tablet between your teeth. It will dissolve in your saliva and produce a pinkish stain. After swishing the stained saliva very thoroughly around and in between your teeth, spit (not wash) it out.
3. Examine your teeth (use a mirror and a good light source) as all the plaque will be stained pink.
4. After toothbrushing as above, re-examine your teeth and remove any residual pink plaque.

These tablets can be used before toothbrushing to help you identify difficult access areas or afterwards to check how well you did. As these tablets tend to also stain the tongue and lips for around two hours, it is advisable not to use these when going out in public.

Vitamin C
Vitamin C powder provides a systemic supplement which will help strengthen the fibres of the gum tissues.

Secondary Gum Conditioning Technique
1. The primary technique cleans the gum tissues on the outside and inside of your teeth. This accounts for 50 per cent of the gum's surface.
2. For the other 50 per cent, which runs between your teeth, use the following combination of little bottle brushes and dental tape:

Back Teeth – Once again, keeping them dry for maximum effectiveness, use inter-dental brushes to both gently massage the gums and clean between the back teeth (the brushes will bend with excess pressure).

Front Teeth – Prior to any bone loss and subsequent gum shrinkage, the triangular spaces between the front teeth are normally too small to be accessed with inter-dental brushes. In these circumstances, use dental floss to clean out the gum grooves on either side of the gum triangle. Be sure to clean on either side of the triangle as flossing straight down on to its peak tends to traumatize the gum tissue.

Torren's Powder
If gum disease is present, the gum tissues may be too tender to use the above techniques effectively. In these circumstances, try using Torren's Powder, which is a type of gum poultice and can be very effective:
1. Take six teaspoons of baking soda and one teaspoon of salt and blend to produce a fine powdered mix.
2. Place a little of this mixture in an egg cup, pick up a small amount with a wet finger tip and pat it on to your gum tissue.
3. Complete this application to all the tissue around either the top or bottom teeth.
4. Leave in place for around five minutes and then repeat for the other jaw.
5. Repeat this poultice twice each day until the acute inflammation of the gum tissues has settled and then start the above gum conditioning technique.

Conclusion
In this day and age we push ourselves very hard in every area of our lives. That is why taking care of yourself is such an important part of your health and fitness programme. Without it, your body often can't respond fully to whatever activity you choose to do. It is also the one area that can bring you back into balance and is the nucleus from which you can go forward daily into the fray with renewed vigour.

It's a Wrap

7

IT IS ESTIMATED THAT EACH OF US has a minimum of 250 chemicals stored in our bodies. Over time our fat stores become saturated with a smorgasbord of chemicals that we breathe, eat, drink or absorb through our skin. Many of these chemicals are manmade and simply cannot be completely broken down and removed through our expired air (breathing out), perspiration, saliva, urine or bowel movements. With each passing year it is becoming more and more difficult for our bodies to handle the progressive chemical overload we are exposed to daily.

These chemicals were developed some 50 or 60 years ago, but we have no digestive enzymes or defensive antibodies to break them down, and therefore they go to the only place we as humans have to store, which is the fat tissue. And fat is not just our gut or our bottom – our brain is by and large fat. Fat is a tissue in the body that stores and builds up, so once the chemicals go into the fat there is no way for them to come out. Valium, cocaine, etc. is therefore stored in the fat cells as well.

'We are the first generation in the history of the world that has been exposed over a lifetime to synthetic and toxic chemicals in our food, air, water and products we use. Before 1940 everyone lived on organic foods; pesticides weren't invented yet. There were no toxic waste dumps, preservatives in foods, antibiotics, Malathion spray, chlorinated water, tight buildings, aerosol sprays, synthetic carpeting, formaldehyde products, or major cosmetics and perfume industries,' says Dr Alan Scott Levin, Associate Professor of Immunology and Dermatology, University of California School of Medicine.

The effects of chemicals on our bodies have been immense. Too many of us are walking round with poor bowel function and a constant dull headache, craving sugar, junk food and cigarettes. Is it any wonder that we don't feel good? Our bodies can only cope with so much. When the bowel can no longer function properly the overload is shifted to the liver, which in turn has to deal with all of the impurities coming out of the intestines. This can produce a knock-on stress effect with all the other organs being affected detrimentally.

Understanding how to limit your exposure to toxins and regularly cleanse your system is vital. If you know about the substances that you are exposed to on a daily basis, you may be able to implement simple but effective changes in your food, personal care products and home environment. If you do have an occasional 'blowout' and toxically overload your system, your body will be able to handle it. But, as it stands, 90 per cent of people are having blowouts on a daily basis, which affects every system in their body.

Breaking down toxins and other chemicals is not possible by losing weight and aerobic exercise alone. So many people don't achieve the desired results from their workouts and the reason is usually this: elimination of toxins from the body must be equal to (or greater than) the input.

It is imperative that you understand how many toxins are entering your environment and your system daily. For instance, the majority of lead we are exposed to comes from the grids of the pavement outside. It is estimated that you would reduce 40 per cent of lead consumption by simply removing your shoes at the door. Most of us solely associate lead with pipes and naïvely assume that if we do not have lead pipes in our homes we are not being exposed. This obviously is not the case. In addition to lead being tracked into the home, several other toxins accumulate on the bottom of our shoes, some of which have been banned for years.

Chemical Scaffolding

Every year an estimated 400 million tons of chemicals are produced and approximately a thousand new substances developed. In addition to knowing little about the long-term effects of each individual chemical, even less is known about the risks associated with exposure to a cocktail of these chemicals. Vyvyan Howard, a foetal toxico-pathologist at Liverpool University and member of the government's Advisory Committee on Pesticides, points out that 'We don't have the tools to analyze how mixtures of these chemicals work, and we probably never will. To test just the commonest 1,000 toxic chemicals in combinations of three would require at least 166 million different experiments. But when we do look, we find surprising interactions. The only logical way forward is to reduce exposure as much as possible.'

A study conducted by a group of scientists at Exeter University's Greenpeace laboratory in 2003 discovered a total of 35 hazardous chemicals in house dust that belonged to one of five groups of chemicals, all known to be carcinogenic, toxic or damaging to either the reproductive function or the immune system. Additional tests revealed a further 140 other chemicals in the dust including flame-retardants, solvents and petrol additives.

Obviously, our homes are not the only source of the toxins that are accumulating in our bodies. The products that we bring into our home have a large impact as well. Common offenders are bleach, washing-up liquid, air fresheners and washing powder as well as glass, mirror and window cleaners. Effects can be obvious such as itchy eyes, headache, nausea, disorientation and skin rashes — or the effects can be more subtle and at the same time more profound, damaging the central nervous system and the immune system, liver and lungs. Less considered and equally as toxic are personal care products.

Our lotions, shower gels, soaps, cosmetics, shampoos, deodorants, toothpastes and mouthwashes all contain a plethora of chemicals. Shockingly, the cosmetics and toiletries sector remains self-regulated. This means that individual companies are responsible for testing their products and it is up to their employed experts to decide if they are safe. The result is that over 9,000 chemicals are regularly used in the cosmetics industry. Again, while there are banned ingredients, and those which have been deemed harmful can only be used in small enough quantities to comply with health and safety regulations, the long-term consequences of these substances remains a mystery. Scientists have shown that an estimated 8–10,000 toxins are potentially absorbed through the skin from commercial cosmetics and toiletries. An unsettling thought when most of us use between six and 12 personal care products daily.

It is important to note here that (unlike in the food industry) in the cosmetics and toiletries industry labels of 'organic' and 'natural' can refer to as little as one per cent of the product (which means the 'organic' or 'natural' ingredients being emphasized to sell the product may well be virtually non-existent). The Food Standards Agency has the authority to regulate the use of the term 'organic' on our food products and ensure that they contain at least 95 per cent organic ingredients, but its power does not extend outside the food industry.

Don't be deceived therefore by the terms 'natural' or 'organic' on toiletries and cosmetics, and always read the labels. Just because you are in a 'natural' shop or department doesn't mean that you will be purchasing all natural products. Manufacturers continue to incorporate chemical substances such as mineral oils and petrochemicals as they are cost-effective, not prone to oxidization and have a guaranteed shelf life of up to three years or more. The addition of synthetic fragrances and artificial colours in products are based on attracting the consumer and assist with disguising putrefaction and rancidity. Fortunately, there are an increasing number of quality products available today that are environmentally friendly and less toxic.

We can't forget that included in our toxic exposure and overload is the chemicals that we ingest through eating. Toxic chemicals get into the environment by being sprayed on crops, running off into our water supply, are absorbed by fish and other animals that eat the crops or swim in the water, until they finally turn up on our plate in the form of meat, fish and eggs. The toxic overload becomes more concentrated the further up the food chain you go. And, as we are at the top of the food chain, we get the full onslaught of this toxic build-up.

Toxins are also prevalent in our food in the form of additives, preservatives, artificial sweeteners and flavour enhancers. There are 540 food-additive compounds that are deemed safe by the regulatory agencies. Included in the list for the UK are additives banned in other countries. Clearly, with countries in disagreement about which additives are safe and in what quantity, it leaves the consumer with no clear guidelines.

Also startling is the fact that it is not mandatory to test the safety of food flavourings. Flavourings are only controlled on a case-by-case basis if they are proved to be harmful. Erik Millstone, reader in science policy at the University of Sussex, points out that 'Most food additives were approved many years ago before test data had to be made public. Most of the data was industry information reviewed by people who were paid consultants to the food industry. You cannot say it is independent.'

For more in-depth information order 'Chemicals in Products: Safeguarding the Environment and Human Health' by the Royal Commission on Environmental Pollution. It is published by The Stationery Office and available from www.tso.co.uk/bookshop or by phoning 0870 6005522.

So, what is a person to do? In an ideal world we would live in a pollution-free environment, eat untainted foods and drink pure water. However, that isn't going to happen (especially as we all love a little bit of poison). What we can do is to keep pollutants to a minimum by eliminating toxic household cleaners and personal care products, as well as periodically getting rid of our toxins through a detoxification programme.

I understand that the thought of overhauling all of your cleaning supplies and toiletries can be overwhelming to say the least. But I will pass on to you some practical tips and my list of favourite products to help make the task a bit easier for you.

In Your Face!

When we walk into the beauty section of the large department stores it is so easy to be seduced by the advertising banners proclaiming miracles in jars, hopes and dreams in creams and magic potions in their lotions. It's been a very long time, probably 20 years, since I bought a skin product for myself in a department store, having learnt about all the ingredients used in the brands. I've always kept it simple but never really found anything natural that I was in love with until I came across two aestheticians, Fiona and Marie, who have their own practice in London.

I was incredibly impressed with Fiona and Marie's no-nonsense attitude and knowledge and fell in love with a product they recommend called Environ. What I learnt from Fiona and Marie is the following:

Within the skin care/cosmetic industry, companies can make claims for their products with very little or no scientific fact to back them up. The image of the woman with flawless skin advertising the product is rarely pictured showing us what her skin looked like before. It was very likely flawless then. We should be told the age of the person. How often are products for mature skin shown alongside a picture of a young woman? Cross-section diagrams of the skin can make it all look very scientific, yet where is the data to accompany the diagram?

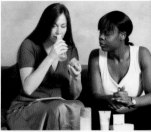

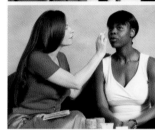

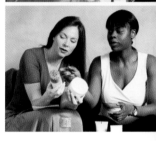

Having gone through Jocelyn's hair, skin and body products, which are full of petrochemicals and other unwanted ingredients, Carole shows Jocelyn the more desirable alternative products.

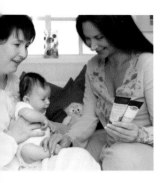

Like most mothers, Ghislaine was using well-known baby products which contained harmful chemical ingredients. Carole shows Ghislaine all the alternatives, from nappy rash cream to non-steroidal eczema cream, bath products and other non-pharmaceutical applications, as well as nappies and clothing.

How many people was it tested on, how old were they, how long did they use it for and what was their skin like before?

For example, a product may promise to be a 'seven-day wrinkle remover' but that is simply not possible – it takes six weeks for the skin to go through just one skin cycle. What that means is that it takes six weeks for a new skin cell to be produced in the basal layer, to mature and make its way to the surface. The wrinkle has taken years to appear – it cannot disappear in a week.

We are also met with banners advertising ingredients that have become household names, for example retinols and collagen. Beware: the amount of active ingredient is often minute. Therefore it has very little effect at a cellular level. The collagen molecule is too large to pass through the skin and can only stay on the surface, nourishing the dead skin cells we are about to shed.

These days one of the advances in skin health has been brought about by the merging of pharmaceuticals and cosmetics companies to produce what is now known as cosmeceuticals. These are products that promote 'skin health', and have active ingredients that can penetrate right down to the basal layer and produce healthier and normalized skin cells.

Because these products have active ingredients it is essential to have a proper skin consultation with a specialist who has been trained in the use of these products. This will minimize any side effects and get you to optimum skin health in the quickest and safest fashion. These products, if sold over-the-counter, could be used inappropriately; for example using the stronger product before you have got your skin used to lower levels of the active ingredients in the milder products could cause problems. People, particularly with problem skin, therefore need a personal consultation with a trained aesthetician, and in Marie and Fiona's practice people are often referred from a dermatologist or plastic surgeon.

In this particular field a lot of the research is being led by plastic surgeons and dermatologists who understand what ingredients are good for the skin and our system, and which contribute to skin health. They therefore don't use parabens, petrochemicals, or other harmful substances.

If cosmetic companies were forced in their advertisements to name their ingredients, how many women would opt for a pot of petrochemicals? How many men and women actually look at the ingredients or even know what they mean?

What You Need To Look For On The Packaging

First, be aware of the terms: for example, hydra-system – is this referring to water or hydration? In the main they are madeup terms which sound vaguely scientific, add a little bit of mystery, but don't mean very much.

Think twice about what the word 'natural' actually means. This does not necessarily mean safe or harmless. There are lots of natural products and plant products that can cause side effects. One example would be alpha hydroxy acids. These products, which are derived from sugarcane and fruit acids, can cause redness and irritation of the skin.

Check how much vitamin A is in the product. This may appear on the packaging as retinol, retinol palmitate or retinyl acetate – all of these are vitamin A derivatives. What really matters is how much is in the product. Unfortunately, many products waving the 'retinol' banner have such small amounts in them that they can have very little – if any – effect on the skin.

Look out for animal extracts. This is exactly what it says it is – no thank you, we'll do without this one.

Lastly, when it comes to ingredients remember that they are listed with the largest component first.

CASE STUDY – FACE CREAM STORY

A 37-year-old woman came in to have her lips enhanced with one of the dermal fillers and Marie noticed her skin was very congested.

Marie asked what she was using and the lady replied that she used a particularly expensive product. Marie asked if she was happy with the way her skin looked. She said yes except for her forehead, cheeks and chin, which were congested. So, basically there was very little of her skin she was actually happy with. Marie asked the obvious question: why was she using a product if she wasn't happy with the results? The lady's answer was because it's the best and it's so beautifully packaged.

Marie then said she had a 'yes or no' question – do you like your skin as it is? The answer was no. So the face cream is not giving you the results that you want Marie concluded – the lady looked at Marie and finally realized that no, it wasn't!

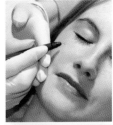

(Below) Fiona Collins doing a Veinwave treatment, which is a simple and effective treatment for broken veins.

If sticking your hand in the fire hurts, stop doing it! Watch out for people who offer what often seems like the obvious solution. For example, people with dry skin are often given very rich products. This can make the skin lazy and stop it producing its own natural moisturiser. Similarly people with oily skin are given oil-free moisturiser and cleansing products that strip the skin of all its oil. This can cause your own oil-producing cells to work overtime to produce more oil and before you know it's a vicious circle. What you need is a product that is going to normalize your sebaceous glands – and kickstart them into producing the right amount of oil.

You will never find that Fiona and Marie have a face cream on special offer. This is because each client needs to be treated as an individual with individual needs. They therefore have a variety of ranges and a variety of products within each range to suit each individual. One size does not fit all – there are different products for people with mature skin, acne, dry, oily or combination skin, rosacea etc.

In Fiona and Marie's opinion, Crème de la Mer and La Prairie should not be used by anyone under the age of 35 as it is generally too rich for them and causes congestion. But they do look good on the dressing table...

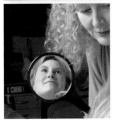

(Above) Aesthetician Marie Duckett advising a new client on what specific treatments and products would work for her.

Don't Be Seduced

Fiona – dressed up to the nines – visited several department stores where she was steered towards the more expensive ranges by sales staff keen to make a commission. She then visited them again; this time dressed casually, and was encouraged to buy the cheaper ranges, if she got any attention at all.

Expensive does not always mean better. Ask lots of questions as to why the product is being recommended. You do not want answers such as 'it's lovely' or 'it smells wonderful'. Fiona and Marie believe in trying before buying and are always happy to hand out samples – something that department stores very rarely do unless they need to get rid of stock or are promoting a specific brand. Stores often don't develop relationships with their clientele – they only care for you as long as you are in front of them and then it's on to the next client.

Normal skin can get away with having most products used on it, but anyone that has any kind of problem skin needs more specialized care. A visit to a dermatologist is not usually necessary for day-to-day skin problems as dermatologists are mainly interested in diseases of the skin and not general skin care. A good aesthetician will always know if your skin problem is beyond their area of expertise and would know who to refer you to.

There are lots of men with pockmarks and acne scars because years ago young boys were not given adequate help with skin problems. So let's not fail them now. Women need to look at their sons, husbands or partners – they need skin care too. Men have ingrowing hairs, blackheads, shaving rash, poor skin texture and rosacea. They also need protection against all the free radicals, the thinning ozone layer and pollution.

The marketing of most products is aimed at women – the glossier the nicer – but it doesn't mean it works the best. Advertising and products should be more asexual and brochures should indicate in simple non-scientific language how products actually work.

Years ago there was a huge difference between the quality of cheaper and more expensive products – but this has now narrowed. Why does it cost £370 for a jar of La Prairie moisturiser? What does it have in it to make it so expensive? What do you get for £135 from Crème de la Mer? According to the sales person, it is full of natural ingredients that, amazingly, can work differently on different skin types, leaving each one energized, dewy and brighter ... and it will diminish open pores, fine lines and wrinkles. Fiona and Marie do not agree.

CASE STUDY – LINDA'S STORY

Everything on Linda's dressing table cost the earth. Because she was spending so much on her products and because she read so many 'advertorials' she was convinced she was doing the best by her skin. On examination, however, her skin was dull and lifeless. We convinced her to try a range we believe in called Environ, which is based on vitamins. She is now a complete convert and her skin care costs half of what it used to. It doesn't look glamorous on the dressing table but it has made her skin look and feel vibrant and healthy.

If you have a quiet half hour one day, why don't you telephone the big department stores and ask to be put through to one of the cosmetic counters?

Ask them what is in their moisturiser. Ask what it can do for your skin and why you should try it. While the salesperson is talking write down the key words she uses and look at them when you hang up. You will discover that most of the adjectives used are nice words like 'dewy', 'energized', 'vibrant', 'refined' and so on. Unfortunately you will not hear a lot about what exactly a product can do, and the data from clinical trials supporting their claim.

Good products for skin care do exist. For example, Jane Iredale Mineral Make-up sells foundation, concealers, translucent powder and sunblock with no petrochemicals, no preservatives and no artificial colouring which allows the skin to breathe on its own. Therefore there is less chance of getting blackheads or blemishes and less chance of a sensitivity reaction because there are no chemicals. This is true for any authentic natural range of products.

In department stores you test make-up on the back of your hand. Fiona and Marie believe in testing on your face – the place you will be wearing it! They send people away with the make-up on to see if they like it in natural light. If they are happy they will come back.

Another question they ask their clients is if they have a drawer containing all the products they have bought that didn't suit them. Invariably the answer is yes ... and the average drawer contains about £300 worth of products.

Contact Fiona and Marie on 020 7908 3773 or at fionamarie@ukonline.co.uk for Environ and Jane Iredale Mineral Make-up

Special Products By Special People

When the first natural skin products appeared on the market they left a lot to be desired. More often than not their scents were noxious, they felt heavy and tacky once applied and the packaging was unappealing. Now, not only can they compete with known brands that sell in our chemists and department stores, the quality and integrity far surpass them.

Just because a product is sold in a health food shop or in the so-called natural sector of a department store, does not guarantee that it is free of all artificial ingredients. You have to check the labels and, if possible, smell the product. If you don't like the smell, I believe that it's not for you. Feeling the product is another way for you to be sure that it is suitable for you. The shelf lives of these products are far less than what you are used to, and that's a good thing. Half the ingredients put into your standard cosmetics are what allow these goods to last for years.

When choosing your products it is a good idea to have a few alternatives for your body, face and hair. This way your system won't tire of your purchases and you will be able to adapt to your skin's needs as they can change according to season and climate, monthly cycles, toxicity, energy levels and health status.

Another recommendation when you are starting out is to choose scent-free or citrus-type smells as they tend to be more cleansing orientated. The reason for this is that if you are adapting your food and exercise regimes and doing an overall clean out then your sense of smell will alter. It is likely that the scents you have been attracted to will become sickly or repugnant, and you want as little interference as possible while clearing out your system.

Smell is very personal and many of us are unaware of how we actually smell to other people. Also, if the scent that you are wearing is sweet or pungent, conditions such as headaches, disorientation, sinus problems and irritated skin may be aggravated by your chosen smell. Try having a month without your usual scent.

As lovely as essentials oils are, they can distract and irritate any detox, so think twice when you treat yourself to a facial or massage or warn your therapist that you want fragrance-free organic oils and products. If, as is more often the case than not, they cannot accommodate your request, ask if you can take in your own products. I keep a bag of essentials in my car for any eventuality so if I stay the night somewhere or go to the gym or a spa I'm never caught out.

What's the point of having a facial or body treatment if it's just going to put rubbish back into your system? If you are just about to protest about how fantastic your regular treatments are, remember it's not due to the product as much as the actual application, massage and relaxing ambiance. You don't have to forgo any of that, just change your product choice.

Whenever I travel, apart from Environ and Circaroma, I take a choice of organic oils from Bioceuticals plus a few of their essential oils and their pure royal jelly face cream, as well as Bharti Vyas's face balm. I and my colleagues have tried hundreds of creams and find that nine out of 10 aggravate the skin and a breakout ensues. Whatever you choose make sure you don't drown your skin in it as your pores will not benefit – less is more. When it comes to eyes, don't take the oil or crème directly around the rim as that causes puffiness – just apply moisturizer to the cheek bone directly under the eye.

For manicures and pedicures there is at last an alternative to the heavily used mineral oil, petroleum and paraben-based products that we have used for decades (and which can easily be compared to heavy duty household cleaners that require you to wear rubber gloves when using.)

Product Recommendations

Every product range that we are recommending here has been tried and tested by myself and the LifeSmart team – as well as hundreds of clients over the years. They are appropriate for men, women and children with special sections in some ranges for babies, children and men. Also worth mentioning are the deodorants provided by some of the following brands which are all made from natural, clean ingredients. Green People have an effective natural crystal spray and roll-on. If you like something scented, the Organic Pharmacy do an excellent deodorant.

All the following products are available worldwide and through the Internet. All phone numbers given are for the UK unless indicated otherwise, so if you are calling from outside the UK you will need to dial 00 44 first and drop the first zero.

YOUR BATHROOM CABINET

A'kin by the Purist Company

A'kin skincare uses the purest organic ingredients, chosen for their skin-friendly compatibility. They are carefully crafted into highly effective formulations designed to give you maximum benefit for your individual skin needs. All A'kin products are free from sulfates, ethoxylates, parabens, propylene glycol, petrochemicals, silicones and artificial colours. A'kin products are organic, vegan, 100 per cent natural botanical aromatherapy and formulated without animal ingredients or animal testing.

Will Evans is the Technical Director of the Purist Company, an Australian company that created and manufactures the A'kin range. Will is a specialist cosmetic chemist whose lifetime's work has been concerned with the function and safety of cosmetic ingredients. Over the course of his studies he uncovered that virtually all cosmetic/toiletry products on the market use ingredients that contain so-called 'objectionable trace impurities' or known toxins and carcinogens. This led him to develop the ultra-pure A'kin products.

Will is a self-styled consumer/industry advocate, involved in submissions to the Australian Ingredient Disclosure Regulations Committee. Will believes that the current regulations are flawed to the detriment of consumers and upholds a 'truth in labelling' ethic. He encourages consumers to air their concerns, in a hope that the industry will recognize the need for change.

Tel: 0207 504 8099
www.purist.com

Barefoot Botanicals

Help is at hand for sufferers of dry, sore and irritated skin with the S.O.S. range from Barefoot Botanicals. Safe and gentle for even the most sensitive skins, the 100 per cent plant-derived S.O.S. products are packed with natural soothing essential oils and botanical extracts.

All the products are gentle enough to be used every day by every member of the family, including babies and children. While good for generally itchy, sore and dry skin, people with eczema and psoriasis can also use the S.O.S. range. It brings relief to those who have used harsh, chemical-ridden steroid creams. Six products are available in the S.O.S. line including: Skin Rescue Moisturizing Body Wash, Intensive Skin Rescue Cream, Intensive Skin Rescue Bath Oil, Foot Rescue Balm, Hair and Scalp Rescue Shampoo and Hair and Scalp Rescue Conditioner.

Barefoot Botanicals creates unique products from blends of botanical extracts, vitamins and pure essential oils. They are 100 per cent plant origin, GM-free and free of animal products, synthetic perfumes, preservatives and colours. The founders, Jonathan Stallick and Hilery Dorrian, are both practicing homeopaths.

Barefoot Botanical products are available at Harrods, Fresh & Wild, Planet Organic and health food shops.

Tel: 0870 220 2273
www.barefoot-botanicals.com

Bestcare Products Ltd

Bestcare sources Original Himalayan Crystal Salt, which has the world's highest elemental content with 84 of the nutritional elements we need. It is used for rejuvenating, bathing, replenishing the skin, drinking therapy and flavouring food. It contains no impurities from environmental pollution. It can be beneficial for a host of ailments from athlete's foot to menopause and arthritis to psoriasis. It also balances the body's pH factor and gets rid of heavy metals such as lead, mercury and arsenic.

Orgon provides complementary products that alkalize your system using plant-derived minerals and a ph value of 8.5. They include a herbal tea, a fortifying vegetable foodstuff that can be added to cereal, juices and yoghurt. They complete the range with a vitalizing hair tonic, Alkabath alkaline bath salts as well as face and body care products which can be used for soaking in, massage, dental care, genital and anal care and face peeling.

Bestcare also supplies the Original Tuebinger Amalgam Blocker Toothpaste. Brushing one's teeth with an ordinary toothpaste causes the emission of mercury to increase by 5-10 times, returning to the original level of emission only after 1-2½ hours. In contrast, brushing with Original Tuebinger Toothpaste has a long-term minimizing effect on the emission of mercury and mercury vapour and can even prevent it completely.

In addition Bestcare provides the Robert Gray Intestinal Cleansing Program™. Robert Gray is a nationally known nutrition counsellor and Director of the Food for Health Institute. He is also a professional member of the American Association of Nutritional Consultants and the American Herb Association. Most of the (unhealthy) foods eaten today form mucoid (slimy) substances in the intestinal tract. These then accumulate into a build-up of stagnant matter in the intestines. This matter can block proper elimination, inhibit proper absorption of nutrients and serve as a breeding ground for germs and parasites. The result is a pollution of blood and lymph and thereby a poisoning of the entire system. This causes a chronic drain on health and vitality that seems normal to too many. However, it is possible with the Robert Gray Intestinal Cleansing Program™ to remove this accumulation of stagnant waste material, which otherwise would never leave the bodies of most people. Many people have experienced extensive improvements in vigour, vitality and overall health.

Tel: 01342 410 303
www.bestcare-uk.com

Burt's Bees

Burt's Bees' first 'factory' was an abandoned one-room school house in Maine. The company sold bottled honey and beeswax stove, furniture and shoe polish at craft fairs around Maine. By 1992, they were making half a million beeswax candles a year. The company is now based in North Carolina and sells their products globally.

Burt's Bees offers an extensive range of products including: bath and body care, skin care, cosmetics, natural hair care, hand and foot care, men's grooming, baby care, natural remedies, and travel and sample kits. I highly recommend their cuticle cream.

www.burtsbees.com

Circaroma

If I was going to give an award for packaging and best use of essential oils Circaroma would be up there in the top two. As well as a full range of face and body products there is a fabulous range of candles that are not overpowering and are all contained beautifully within a glass jar and lid. Their skincare embodies the sensation of pure aromas linking mind and body. They also make exclusive products for a few choice spas.

Circaroma was founded by aromatherapist Barbara Scott. It has a simple philosophy, which is to use only the finest natural and organic skincare ingredients available that work in harmony with your skin. They do not use any synthetic ingredients such as mineral oils, parabens, sulphates, artificial aromas or colours, which they believe can adversely affect the health of your skin.

Circaroma skincare will appeal to your senses through aroma and touch allowing you to care for your skin with exceptionally pure ingredients in high performance and simple, effective skin formulas. Circaroma Rose Hand Cream was recently named Best Hand Cream in the best-selling book *21st Century Beauty Bible*, beating a number of world-famous brands.

Barbara believes you can care for your skin in a genuinely natural way while achieving effective results and experiencing beautiful aromas. She started experimenting with organic ingredients in the kitchen of her London home and selling bespoke products to her clients. Her success led her to develop her small range further and she began selling to the public on a stall at Spitalfields Organic Market in London. Encouraged by the huge interest in her products, she set up Circaroma in January 2000. Today Circaroma products are still produced in small batches and Barbara employs only qualified aromatherapists and herbalists to produce the products.

Tel: 0207 359 1135
www.circaroma.com

Desert Essence

Desert Essence was the first Tea Tree Oil company in America and offers a purist approach to therapeutic natural beauty with every product. Desert Essence continues to expand into new categories and offers facial, oral (excellent dental floss), hair and body care products with shea butter, jojoba oil and aromatherapy oils. They produce excellent deodorants, skin care products and spot treatment.

Desert Essence is available at health food shops.

Energys Sun Love

Sun Love is a natural, gentle approach to being in the sun. It can be applied over your daily moisturizer, under make-up, or on the whole body during sensible periods of sunbathing. This is not a sunblock! Sun Love provides natural melanin (the body's own tanning agent) from sunflowers to support natural tanning.

It also provides the sun-protective antioxidants green tea, rutin, vitamins A and E and co-enzyme Q10, highly protective Argan oil (from Morocco), MSM, aloe vera and willowherb, plus regenerative, nurturing and moisturizing factors including nano-lipids filled with pulp of sea buckthorn (rich in vitamin C) and starflower oil (rich in GLA). Use sparingly. Sun Love also carries energy resonance encoded on the absolute of Pink Lotus and the essential oils of Lemon Scented Tea Tree and Camphor to harmonize the body's energy field. Sun Love contains no titanium dioxide or other chemical or mineral sunblock agents, sodium lauryl sulphate, PEG emulsifiers, propylene glycol, chemical dyes, synthetic fragrances or chemical preservatives, and is not tested on animals.

www.auravita.com

Essential Care

Essential Care creates truly natural personal care with organic and biodynamic plant ingredients. Their special interest is in caring for sensitive and eczema-prone skin. Essential Care is approved under the Soil Association standards, which means all personal care products are 95 per cent organic, eco-friendly and, above all, kind to the skin. It is a unique way for consumers to be assured that the products do not contain any of the following: artificial fragrance or colour, cocamide DEA, lanolin, mineral oil, paraben preservatives, petroleum derivatives, polysorbates, propylene glycol or sodium laureth sulphate. Essential Care believes that there is a link between the widespread use of these substances in products and the rise in skin allergies such as eczema.

Organic personal care is not only more compatible with allergy-prone skin, it is also more effective on all skin. Cold-pressed natural plant oils have a higher vitamin content and nourish and moisturize much more than synthetic preparations. The makers have formulated all of Essential Care's products to provide optimum therapeutic benefit by researching aromatherapy and herbal medicine for over 25 years.

In March 2003, Essential Care's Shampoo was the first ever to be certified with the Soil Association, which is the strictest certifying body in the world for organic health and beauty products. Only five or so companies have achieved their standards for skincare, and Essential Care is the first and only company to have a certified organic shampoo.

The company continues to make its products by hand with over 50 different species of organic herbs and flowers to ensure that her high-quality standards are met. Based in Suffolk, the heart of Essential Care is a small family team of Margaret, Colin and daughter Abi.

Tel: 01284 728 416
www.essential-care.co.uk

Green People

Green People was launched in 1997 with the aim of offering highly effective organic formulations made from 100 per cent gentle ingredients. They research, develop, formulate and manufacture their hand-made health and beauty formulations in-house. Green People does not use any irritating emulsifiers, harsh foaming agents, or any of the unnecessary synthetic additives common in many of today's health and beauty products.

Proof Magazine rated Green People's Sun Lotion 'Excellent' in 2002. It is more than 84 per cent organic, combines natural UVA and UVB filters with antioxidants to support the skin's immune system and helps protect against cell damage. Green People also offer an SPF15 Lotion with Suntan

Accelerator which is the first organic sun cream formulation without aluminum or other heavy metals to boost your body's ability to tan. The suntan accelerator is a mixture of vitamin B2 (riboflavin) and the amino acid tyrosine. These stimulate the formation of melanin (our own natural sunscreen) in your skin which promotes a quicker tan and additional protection.

Green People grew out of Charlotte Vohtz's desire to help her daughter, Sandra, who had severe eczema and allergies. Charlotte highly recommends the 'Hawthorn and Artichoke Formula' obtained from leading international herbalists at The College of Phytotherapy, as well as a daily dose of organic omega-3 and omega-6 essential fatty acids for anyone suffering from similar symptoms.

Green People offers an exclusive range of pure, organic ingredients just for men which includes facial care, shaving and hair and body products.

One of the most impressive parts of their range is the comprehensive babies and children's products.

Green People products and supplements can be found at health food shops.

www.greenpeople.co.uk

Jason Organics

The Jason brand, which was founded in the US in 1959, promises to give consumers an alternative choice to mass market, chemically dependent products. The core value of this visionary company is to offer natural products containing pure, nutritional and organic ingredients that deliver topical benefits to the skin, hair and body. Jason makes all of their own products in their own factory and always have (most cosmetics companies don't do this). They have spent the last 45 years developing their philosophy and helping people with their personal care and beauty needs at reasonable prices. Jason proves that being organic doesn't mean it needs to be expensive. Their facilities are licensed by the FDA, certified organic, and operate at a pharmaceutical level of quality.

Jason's vast range of organic toiletry products are devoid of mineral oils, petrolatum PABA, isopropyl, alcohol, propylene, glycol, aluminum chlorohydrate and sodium laureth sulphate.

There are no artificial colours or animal byproducts and the packaging is bio-degradable and/or recyclable. All products are certified vegan.

The product range is impressive and has everything consumers may require from head to toe, the best-tasting oral care, bath products, body lotions and body butter (which are superb). Jason produces a vast range of natural deodorants that have been lauded by the press for the pureness of the ingredients. The toothpaste range is preferred and approved by many homeopaths since it is chalk-free. Jason also offers a wonderful range of products exclusively for men.

Jason's impressive manufacturing plant in California is a Certified Organic Processor and is the first personal care manufacturer to be given this status by the Californian Certified Organic Farmers Certification. The company is also an active member of the Organic Trade Association. There are major plans for UK certification and the US is collaborating with the Soil Association to make this happen.

Jason products are available from Harrods, Selfridges, John Bell & Croyden and other health food shops.

Tel: 020 7435 5911

Lavera

Lavera began with Thomas Haase, who as a child suffered from neurodermatitis. He found that conventional cream brought no relief, so from an early age he took an active interest in ingredients and alternative skin care options. As a student he opened a health food shop, cultivated plants and produced herbal extracts to develop his first formulations.

After working for 10 years on developing cosmetics, Thomas started Lavera. Today Lavera is a small, family company that employs over 80 people at its own premises near Hanover, Germany.

Lavera offers a skin and body care range specifically for men that have been especially formulated for sensitive skin including: shaving cream, aftershave lotion, a shower shampoo and deodorant.

Lavera was the first manufacturer worldwide to produce a 100 per cent mineral-based sun protection. The formulas for adults, children and babies start protecting instantly after application. Lavera's sun protection products provide protection against UVA, UVB and UVC rays. Lavera offers special products for individual sun protection needs and insect repellent. It also offers the first natural self-tanning lotion, as well as aftersun with scientifically proven effective moisturizing factor.

Lavera sells a wonderful range of natural cosmetics in addition to their skin care line. It has grown out of the demand for controlled natural cosmetics with visible results. Their range of sensitive, decorative cosmetics includes: face powder, concealer, rouge, lipgloss, lip pencils, lipstick, eye liner, eye shadow and mascara.

Lavera products are available at Oliver's of Kew, Organic Pharmacy, Here in Chelsea Farmer's Market, Nelsons Homeopathic Chemist, Fresh & Wild, Planet Organic, and other health food shops and pharmacies.

www.lavera.co.uk

The Little Herbal Company

The Little Herbal Company is a true cottage industry. The founder, Lesley Robinson, started the company in 1999 after returning from a holiday in Zimbabwe. While in Zimbabwe Lesley was in constant pain due to a knee injury. Medication was having no effect, so their guide took her to see the local witch doctor, Roseanna. Within two days Lesley managed to walk 14km without painkillers. Roseanna's herbal medicine had worked miracles on her knee. The rest as they say is history. Lesley gave up her job as a clinical marketing manager with a pharmaceutical company and committed herself to making a few of Africa's healing remedies available in the UK.

Themba is a wonderful skin cream for treating psoriasis, eczema, itchy or dry skin and spots. It is a combination of the active ingredient from the African Kigelia or sausage tree – a known remedy for skin problems – with antiseptic lavender and soothing aloe. The African Shona translation for Themba is 'hope'.

Simba, derived from the African potato, provides natural immune support. Scientists at St James's Hospital in Leeds have done laboratory tests that show this supplement increases production of the body's fighter cells, boosting the immune function. It can be particularly effective for treating conditions such as chronic fatigue syndrome, MS, lupus and ME. The African Shona translation for Simba is 'strength'.

Kuswera Zuro is a soft, nourishing cream that is described as 'food for your face'. For centuries African women have been admired for their beautiful complexions and have used the African potato in the form of a balm to combat exposure to sun, to limit the effects of ageing and to repair damaged skin. Kuswera Zuro was created using the best combination of African herbal knowledge and Western technology.

A percentage of The Little Herbal Company's profits are donated to help Roseanna's local community in Zimbabwe.

Tel: 01484 685 100
www.littleherbal.co.uk

Lotus Emporium

I came across these stunning products by chance at the Vitality Exhibition. In terms of smell, uniqueness and presentation of their scented bath salts, soaps and incense this company has set a very high standard.

It all started in 1998 when Kate and Jeremy Williams began making candles and incense in a garden shed in Bath. From that time Lotus Emporium has grown and expanded, but the focus remains on the personal touches which emphasize the products' home-made and natural appeal. Kate has developed a small collection of aromatherapy blends that are exclusive to Lotus Emporium and used throughout the range. All her ingredients are wild and organically grown wherever possible. No synthetic colourants, perfume oils or preservatives are used.

Their smudge sticks, incense and native American herbs are sourced from a native American cooperative in New Mexico. All the herbs are wild crafted which means their ingredients have been collected when in season and therefore at their most powerful. Smudging is traditionally used to clear spaces from unwanted negativity whether to do with a person or situation. It's also very soothing. You'll not only find many things to use to pamper yourself, but great gifts for friends and family as well.

Tel: 01225 448 011
www.lotusemporium.co.uk

Louise Galvin Sacred Locks

Louise Galvin offers a range of hair products including a hair moisturizer, hair treatment mask and hair cleanser. I have to say that of all the natural hair products these are my favourite. Louise keeps everything very simple and her products suit all types of hair. She decided that even though she could make more profit by bringing out a different shampoo for each hair problem and condition, it wasn't necessary. There is a reason why two very high-end stores on both sides of the Atlantic (Space NK and Bergdorf Goodman) are selling her products. Word is spreading fast. Louise has also brought out a hand and body wash, as well as a travel version of her hair products.

Tel: 0207 289 5131
www.louisegalvin.com

Muk'ti Botanicals

Muk'ti Botanicals offers a complete range of facial, body and hair care products. Products use optimal concentrations of pure essential therapeutic grade oils, certified organic herbal extracts, essential fatty acids, natural vitamins and plant-based liposomes that all significantly contribute to moisture retention, oxygenation and cell regeneration. Products are hand-crafted in small batches to ensure quality and freshness. They do not test any of their products on animals, and with the exception of beeswax and honey in only a few of their products, do not use animal-derived ingredients.

Mukti Lloyd, Managing Director and founder, has a Diploma of Applied Science in Remedial Therapies, a Diploma of Beauty Therapy, Cosmetology and Make-up Artistry, a Diploma in Aromatherapy and is currently completing a Bachelor of Science. With first-hand experience as a natural therapist in the beauty and hairdressing industry, the development of the range came about as a response to what was currently available in the market place and her desire to offer truly natural products. Muk'ti

Botanicals offers a comprehensive Therapist Training Manual that includes details on all of their products, a glossary of key ingredients used in their products, as well as a dictionary of toxic ingredients which are included in many other cosmetics and toiletries.

Muk'ti Botanicals are distributed in the UK by Planet Blue.

Tel: 0208 748 9200
www.muktibotanicals.com.au

Natracare

Natracare offers women feminine hygiene products that they can trust and rely upon because they are made by a campaigning and pioneering company that is recognized by the Ethical Society for putting women and the environment first. Natracare's tampons, which were the first all-cotton tampons on the market since the 1940s, are the only fully certified organic cotton tampons from raw cotton. They are fully certified by IMO and the Soil Association.

Founder of Natracare and an environmentalist for more than 25 years, Susie Hewson says, 'Many women are unaware that rayon and rayon-cotton blends are widely used in the manufacture of tampons. Rayon is commonly chlorine-bleached and is fibre for fibre more absorbent than cotton. Dioxin, a byproduct of chlorine bleaching, should be a real concern for women, as it is linked to cancer, endometriosis, low sperm counts and immune suppression even at low levels.' Such is the concern for North American women, that US senators have introduced The Robin Danielson Act (H.R. 373) which directs their Department of Health to conduct research to determine the extent to which the presence of dioxin, synthetic fibres and other additives in tampons and related products pose any health risks to women including endometriosis and breast, ovarian and cervical cancers. Dioxins are found throughout the environment in varying levels and they have been found to collect in the fatty tissues of animals, including humans. Considering a woman may use as many as 11,000 tampons in her lifetime, she may be subjecting herself to additional dioxin exposure.

Natracare tampons, which are free of herbicides, pesticides and dioxin residuals and are totally chlorine free, have been a major benefit for women since they were first developed back in 1989 as an alternative to the usual available brands. Natracare's sanitary pads and panty shields are natural and over 95 per cent biodegradable. They too provide comfortable, reliable protection without harmful chemicals and synthetics.

Natracare products are available at Fresh & Wild, Planet Organic and Sainsbury's and other health food shops.

www.natracare.com

Naturtint

Naturtint is the first permanent hair colourant without ammonia or resorcinol. Naturtint offers 100 per cent grey cover. Their products carry a full range of colours and use active vegetable ingredients to nourish and repair your hair. Naturtint is against animal testing and is available in selected health food shops.

www.naturesdream.co.uk

On Beauty

On Beauty has combined the finest ingredients known to have anti-ageing properties to protect, nourish and firm your skin. Everyone over the age of 25 loses an amount of naturally occurring collagen in their body, year on year. This can most easily be seen through the formation of lines and wrinkles as the skin loses its elasticity. All On Beauty products are 100 per cent natural and are formulated from the highest-quality ingredients.

The entire proto-Col range is suitable for sensitive skin. My favourite products are their proto-Col Instant Manicure and Instant Pedicure. Both provide a refreshing treat when you need a quick energy boost or a bit of pampering. With anti-ageing antioxidants, pure essential oils and Dead Sea Salts, Instant Manicure will smooth, exfoliate, nourish and rejuvenate your hands in 60 seconds. This gentle massage encourages the essential oils (Rosemary and Peppermint) to sink into the skin's surface and makes your hands look brighter, smoother and revitalized. The Instant Pedicure is a spa-inspired blend of essential oils and

salts to exfoliate and moisturize. Swiss Alps Lavender and Capsicum will ease aches and pains, while Tea Tree Oil keeps fungal infection at bay and Lemongrass acts as an anti-perspirant to keep feet fresh.

Tel: 0870 770 3861 or 0870 770 3860
www.on-beauty.co.uk

Organic Blue

Nominated in 2003 for the 'Best New Non-Food Product' by the Natural Products Industry Awards, Organic Blue offers stylish products of organic quality at excellent prices. Organic Blue's products have been specifically formulated to be therapeutic and offer great performance. It takes the best of ingredients and traditions from around the world – in particular they make available products using many certified organic ayurvedic herbs for the first time in the UK.

Organic Blue offers a range of bodycare, bath and massage oils, vapour/bath mood blends and food supplements. Their bodycare products are certified organic and all other products meet the Soil Association's organic standard. For purity and environmental reasons, where possible, organic quality plants and herbs are used. All products are suitable for both vegetarians and vegans and are not tested on animals.

The idea behind the Organic Blue concept began in late 1999 when the founders spent time trying to find 'natural-quality' products around the world. They felt that no single brand could satisfy all their requirements for depth of products or ingredient quality. Being Indian in origin, yet having grown up in the UK, the founders were becoming aware of how much they were affected in their everyday actions both at home and work by their rich tradition of Jainism – an ancient philosophy based on 'ahimsa' (non-violence) and respect for life.

The founders have been vegetarian since birth, respecting animal life; their grandmother taught them to carefully remove any insect from the house without causing it harm. Hence their attempt to only use products free from animal ingredients. In addition, their mother would often use (and still does) Indian herbs based on ayurvedic recipes to cure them of illnesses, which they accepted as part of the medicinal cabinet. They truly are a fusion of East and West and this is what they have brought to Organic Blue.

Organic Blue products are currently available at larger Sainsbury's and selected health food shops, or by mail order directly from HealthQuest.

Tel: 0208 206 2066
www.organicblue.com

The Organic Pharmacy

The Organic Pharmacy is the first pharmacy to be committed to natural and organic medicines and beauty products. Their products contain no artificial preservatives, pesticides, herbicide residues, mineral oils, petrochemical derivatives, artificial colours or fragrances, harsh detergents, DEA, TEA or PEG derivatives and have not been tested on animals.

Margo Marrone, the creator of the Organic Pharmacy skin care range, believes the quality of the extracts and ingredients used are very important. Instead of using mineral oil, their homeopathic pharmacists prepare all products using organic, cold-pressed vegetable oils of the highest quality. Mineral oil is a byproduct of petrol refinery and is found in almost every major brand. It is used because it is cheap, stable and feels good on the skin, although in fact it suffocates it.

The Organic Pharmacy offers a comprehensive range of skin care, body care, bath, mother and baby care, essential oils, creams and ointments, tinctures and supplements, as well as a complete range of homeopathic remedies. They offer some great kits such as the In-flight Kit, the Quit Smoking Kit, the Surgery Kit and the De-Tox kit. Each of these comes with a handful of products specially chosen to get you or a friend through a less than ideal time. It's also possible to receive award-winning treatments at their clinic and beauty rooms.

The Organic Pharmacy is able to provide service and solutions to all modern problems. They provide professional advice and are excellent at providing alternatives to GP prescriptions, antibiotics or over-the-counter medications. The goal is to provide thoughtful combinations so that your body isn't overloaded.

Margo is a trained pharmacist and homeopath. While pregnant with her daughter, she read an article that talked about carcinogens and toxins in skin care and how we absorb them through our skin. With the dawning realization that the cosmetic industry is one of the least regulated industries and uses all sorts of toxins (including many in shops labelled 'organic'), she set about formulating and making her own products. This was the beginning of the Organic Pharmacy skin care range and eventually the Organic Pharmacy itself. Margo's goal was to create a place where people could come not just for pure and clean products, but also to get professional advice on alternative treatments for common ailments.

Tel: 0207 351 2232

www.theorganicpharmacy.com

Tom's of Maine

For more than 30 years, Tom's of Maine has been creating safe, effective products sourced in nature. Although the company has grown hugely, they continue 'to be guided faithfully by one simple notion – do what is right for our customers, employees, communities and environment.' Tom's of Maine creates safe, effective, natural products free of dyes, sweeteners and preservatives. They harvest, process and package with respect for natural resources; do not test on animals or use animal ingredients; and donate 10 per cent of profits and 5 per cent of employees' paid time to charitable organizations.

Tom's of Maine produces a wonderful range of oral care products including toothpaste and mouthwash.

Tom's of Maine products are available at health food shops.

www.toms-of-maine.com

The Tongue Cleaner™

Scientific studies show that a major cause of bad breath is odour-causing bacteria on the tongue. Especially during sleep, the tongue accumulates an unpleasant film of bacteria and other compounds. This is why after brushing your teeth, fresh breath is difficult to maintain. Bacteria build up on the tongue and can lead to the formation of dental plaque, which may cause tooth decay, periodontal disease and other oral health problems.

Using The Tongue Cleaner™ promotes fresh breath and helps to prevent oral hygiene problems before they develop. You will experience a fresh feeling in your mouth along with restored taste. Quick and simple to use, it can easily become part of your daily oral care routine.

www.pitrock.com

YOUR MEDICINE CABINET

Ainsworths

Ainsworths offer the largest range of homeopathic remedies in the world. John Ainsworth and two fellow pharmacists who had more than 40 years' experience in making homeopathic remedies founded Ainsworths in 1978. They are honoured to have been appointed as Royal Warrant Holder for their supply of homeopathic medicines to the royal family.

Ainsworths offers a unique range of 'Clearing Collection' Mist Sprays – a range of 'feel good' essence sprays, designed to protect, cleanse and clear 'yourself and anywhere you choose to be.' Each of the distinctive sprays is prepared in 'dosage' strength with flower essences made according to the recommendations and methods of Dr Edward Bach. The Clearing Collection sprays include: Cleanse and Protect, Calm and Strengthen, Ground and Go, and Inner Guidance. Each comes with its own guide to the remedies, 'True Self' exercise and recommendations.

They also offer Recovery Plus, which is a product addressing the limitations of Rescue Remedy. The extremely effective formula combines the existing Recovery Plus+ (Dr Bach's original Rescue Formula) with three additional emergency essences to provide the ultimate 'rescue' product to cope with fear, shock or panic. There is also the equivalent crème for cuts, bruises, stings and bites.

www.ainsworths.com

Allergenics

The Allergenics range was formulated after extensive research and dermatological studies in the field of allergies.

Synthetic preservatives, in particular those often found in soaps, shower gels, shampoos etc, cause many skin allergies. All Allergenics' products are composed of 100 per cent natural non-chemical ingredients,are preservative-free and hypoallergenic. Most importantly they are steroid free.

Allergenics Cream is a soothing anti-flare-up emollient for those with easily irritated, dry, itchy skin conditions such as eczema and psoriasis. Developed to help manage dermatological skin conditions without steroids, it is also perfume- and lanolin-free. Allergenics Cream acts as a protective emollient treatment for all skin types including for babies and infants.

The Allergenics range of products includes creams, shampoo, body wash, baby wash, skin lotion and ointment.

www.allergenics.co.uk

Bausch & Lomb

ReNu Comfort Drips are a preservative-free solution which is recommended for use with all soft contact lenses (including continuous wear). It lubricates, cushions and re-wet lenses during wear.

www.bausch.com

Bioforce

Bioforce produces quality, fresh herb extract tinctures prepared from organically cultivated or wild herbs in Switzerland. No pesticides, insecticides, fungicides or chemical fertilizers are used. Alcohol extraction ensures a good balance of the important elements present in each herb. Stringent control analyses before, during and after processing enables tinctures to be produced of a uniform quality and purity. Tinctures are available for a wide range of conditions.

www.bioforce.co.uk

Citricidal

Citricidal is a natural antiseptic that can be taken orally or applied topically to the skin. It is great to take with you when you travel and can be used for everything from gut infections to washing your hands or cutlery. It is also good for insect bites and cuts. See NutriBiotic (page 212) for more information and products.

Delacet

Delacet is an easy-to-use natural herbal cleanser and repellant for head lice and nits. It is a unique dual-action flower extract known for its outstanding properties and has been used successfully in Europe for over 40 years. Laboratory trials have proven its effectiveness after just one application. Delacet is not a shampoo and is very different from many other available products.

Delacet is prepared from organically grown native European plants. It does not contain any harmful chemicals and is free from artificial preservatives, additives and colours. It does not require detection or prolonged combing. The whole family including pregnant, breastfeeding women and children over one year can safely use it. It has not been tested on animals and is suitable for vegans.

A few years ago there was a small group of parents who firmly believed that nature must hold an answer to the head lice problem. They refused to believe that there was no natural solution to this condition and the only way forward was the nit combing procedure. Following the common sense approach they decided to draw on the experience of countries that have no problem with parasite infestation. The result was the introduction of Delacet to the UK.

Delacet is recommended by the Scottish Parent Teacher Council to all schools in Scotland. It is also available on the NHS — unprecedented recognition for an alternative product.

For more information contact Healthpol on 0208 360 0386. Delacet is available from Suma, Infinity Foods, Queenswood, Marigold, Goodness Foods, GFD, Green City, Perrans and Wholefoods Wholesale.

www.delacet.co.uk

International Flower Essence Repertoire

I met Clare Harvey approximately 20 years ago at a retreat called Middle Piccadilly — it had only a few guests, you did your own washing-up, slept whenever you wanted and had massages lasting up to two hours. Clare looked after us all and guided our time and needs. She introduced me to the magic of The Bach Flower remedies and is today recognized as a world authority on all flower essences. Clare is co-director of the International Flower Essence Repertoire and The International Federation for Vibrational Medicine

The whole family including your pets can use flower essences — they are pure and natural.

Available products include:

Australian Bush Flower Essences — provides unique formulations blended using Australian Bush Flower Essences with rare remedial qualities, which have been ecologically gathered in unpolluted regions of Australia. Flower essences have been described as vibrational therapy that treats emotional health and well-being. Australian Bush Flower Essences professional range of pure botanical Flower Essences are used all over the world to help manage the emotional demands of everyday life. They also do a range of creams and sprays that complement the flower essences.

Indigo Essences — gem and crystal essences made in Ireland by Ann Callaghan and her nephews Ben and Mica. They are made to be particularly helpful to children. They form a rescue kit that will help with children's emotions, such as feeling lonely, being scared, getting stressed in school etc. The names are self-explanatory (e.g. 'happy', 'no fear' or 'sleep easy') and children of almost any age can choose the essences they need by themselves.

Tel: 01428 741 572
www.healingflowers.com

L-Lysine

Next time you have a cold sore or herpes outbreak don't rush to the chemist. Instead, try L-Lysine. L-Lysine provides a wonderful natural alternative that can be applied topically or taken orally to heal cold sores. Lysine is an essential amino acid. This means that the body cannot produce L-Lysine and this important amino acid must be obtained from dietary intake. A deficiency in lysine can contribute to outbreaks of cold sores and herpes. Taking L-Lysine in supplement form can help prevent or heal an outbreak.

Solgar makes a quality L-Lysine supplement that is available at most health food shops.

Nasaleze

Nasaleze is a unique, natural, organic product that works with your body's own defence mechanisms to strengthen your resistance to allergens such as pollen, animal hair and dust mites. Studies have shown that by naturally enhancing nasal mucus, it is possible to filter out allergens so that only clean air reaches the lungs. Nasaleze works by forming an invisible, gel-like mucus lining in the nasal tract, which acts as a filter for dust and germs.

Nasaleze has been shown to reduce hayfever symptoms in just 3–10 seconds, to relieve asthma in most cases in a few hours, and even eczema symptoms have subsided after approximately three weeks of use twice daily. Nasaleze can also be used to provide effective infection protection against germs and cold bugs in airplanes and office environments.

Nasaleze contains no drugs and has no side effects, which means it is 100 per cent safe for all the family, including children and pregnant women. It is a registered Class 1 Medical Device in the EU and sold in 19 countries worldwide.

Tel: 01535 691 756
www.nasaleze.com

NatraBio Arnica Rub

NatraBio® products have been manufactured and sold in leading health food stores and natural supermarkets for over 20 years. Since its inception, NatraBio® has become one of the most respected brands in the natural products industry, dedicated to a deep, philosophical commitment to the science behind homeopathy and natural healing, and the establishment and adherence to strict pharmaceutical quality standards.

The Arnica Rub is an all-purpose cream for active people of all ages who need relief from overexertion or injuries. This fast-absorbing cream penetrates through the skin to help heal muscle, nerve, tendon and blood vessel damage using arnica and other supporting ingredients.

www.natrabio.com

Natto NKCP

Maintaining optimum blood flow has been repeatedly highlighted by the media in recent years as important for anyone living sedentary lifestyles, anyone with an unhealthy heart and blood vessels, and anyone undergoing long periods of inactivity, for example, during long-haul flights. Although drugs like Aspirin are often taken by those concerned about blood flow, they can have damaging side effects, especially when taken long term.

NKCP is extracted from natto, a traditional Japanese food of fermented soybeans that has been renowned for over 2,000 years for its health-giving properties, and specifically its ability to help maintain a healthy blood system. The problem with natto, however, is fourfold: it has a very unpleasant smell and taste; it contains high amounts of vitamin K2 which can interfere with medicines such as Warfarin; the health-giving properties can vary greatly between different natto brands; and it is difficult for Westerners to obtain.

The Japanese developers of NKCP solved these problems by creating a process that allowed for the beneficial properties of natto to be put in tablet form. NKCP gives the body the nutrients it needs to help it safely optimize blood flow without affecting blood clotting.

Tel: 0208 480 1000
www.healthy.co.uk

Natural Immunogenics

People have known for centuries that silver kills germs. Colloidal silver can be used topically or sublingually for a wide range of common maladies including eye infections (pink eye, conjunctivitis, sty), ear infections, nasal infections, mouth and gum infections, colds and flu and sore throats. It can be used topically on cuts, scrapes, burns and infections as well as for urinary tract infections, respiratory infections, vaginal infections, *candida albicans*, traveller's diarrhoea and water purification.

Medically approved silver products are used every day in hospitals and healthcare centres. But for home use, you need to be more careful and selective. Make sure you choose a 10 part per million formulation that consists of ultra-pure water and silver only and has the smallest particle size possible. Look for documentation by the company.

Sovereign Silver has been found to be highly effective at the lowest

dosages. It is available at natural health centres, natural pharmacies and from health professionals.

www.natural-immunogenics.com

Nourish

Nourish was set up in 1998 by Jane Sheldon Clarke after experiencing difficulties in conceiving. Jane set it up with the goal of passing on what she had learned during this time to help other prospective parents who wanted to approach pregnancy in a thoughtful, health-conscious manner, in addition to those who had been struggling to conceive. She developed a Nourish Conception Conditioning Programme – a natural treatment programme designed to improve the reproductive health of both men and women who are trying to conceive.

The programme is designed to be taken by both partners, includes nutritional complexes, herbal tinctures and essential oils, as well as advice on diet, weight and lifestyle factors such as stress and fatigue. Research has shown that, if both partners adopt a pre-conceptual healthcare programme for at least four consecutive months prior to conception, it is possible to have an impact on reproductive outcomes, both in terms of chances of conceiving and the future health of your baby.

The conception conditioners have been carefully formulated to help achieve optimal health for the egg and sperm by providing nutrients vital for conception and your baby's healthy development, giving support to the excretory systems, providing antioxidants to combat harmful free radicals to help protect genetic material in the egg and sperm, maintaining hormonal function, essential to support your pregnancy, assisting digestion and assimilation of nutrients and providing emotional preparation.

The Organic Aromatherapy Massage Oils have been certified by the Soil Association. The Conception Conditioning Organic Herbal Tincture and Organic Vitex Agnus Castus Fruit Extract have been certified by the Organic Farmers and Growers Association.

Nourish also provides a hypnotherapy CD which helps women prepare their mind and bodies for pregnancy. Jane says: 'Because every experience,

memory and fear is stored in our minds, emotions can play a big role in preventing us from conceiving. Hypnotherapy gives women the tools they need to tap into their subconscious, which can affect how our bodies work and even control how our body produces hormones during our cycle. Once in this deeply relaxed state women can deal with and overcome any fears and anxieties associated with pregnancy and labour and feel positive about their natural ability to conceive.'

www.nourish-fertility.com

NutriBiotic

Inspired by the research and recommendations of the world's only two-time Nobel Laureate, Linus Pauling, PhD, NutriBiotic began work in 1981 developing a variety of forms and dosages of vitamin C and other nutrients. NutriBiotic felt that the public should have the best possible variety of the best possible nutrients at the best possible price.

In 1987 NutriBiotic pioneered the process and use of grapefruit seed extract. You will find a range of products containing Citricidal™, including skin cleansers, shower gel and bubble bath, dental gel, deodorant stick, foot powder, multi-purpose liquid concentrate and CapsulesPlus.

In addition, I highly recommend their ear drops, nasal spray and First Aid skin spray.

www.nutribiotic.com

The Organic Pharmacy

The Organic Pharmacy provides wonderful combinations for men, women and children covering everything from rheumatism to *candida albicans*.

See page 209 for further details.

Passion for Life

Snoreeze is an effective natural anti-snoring throat spray that has been proven in clinical trials. It contains a unique combination of essential oils and vitamins that coat the soft tissues in the throat to help stop the vibrations that cause snoring. The easy-to-use throat spray has been proven to be 93 per cent effective in reducing snoring noise. A double blind controlled study found that Snoreeze eliminated snoring altogether in 50 per cent of participants.

Audiclean provides a safer alternative to cotton buds. It is well known that cleaning earwax with a cotton bud, although common practice, is not recommended and can cause long-term damage to the ear canal. Surprisingly in 1999, there were 7,000 cotton bud injuries resulting in hospital treatment. Audiclean provides a safe, natural and clinically proven alternative to using cotton buds for the removal of earwax. It is quick, simple and easy to use. Made from 100 per cent Sea Serum™, an isotonic solution with no preservatives, it can be used in the bath or shower. Audioclean works in three ways: it cleans ears safely and effectively, disperses earwax plugs quickly, and prevents the build up of earwax. Audioclean can be safely used with babies from six months old.

Passion for Life was founded in 1996 by Philip Artus and Alex Duggan as a result of a shared belief in healthy living and a desire to improve the lives of others by providing innovative, effective solutions to everyday health problems.

Passion for Life products are sold in Boots, Holland and Barrett, Moss, Lloyds Chemists, Superdrug and Asda as well as other health food shops.

www.passionforlife.com

PediTech

Peditech kills bacteria that cause foot odour and helps protect against odour returning. PediTech's unique two-step formula helps eliminate foot odour fast. Initially spray on the feet daily for one week to kill the bacteria that causes foot odour. Regular use thereafter can help protect against odour returning.

www.peditech.com

Selectrolytes

Selectrolytes is a concentrate of electrolytes: sodium, potassium, magnesium, phosphate, chloride and bicarbonate in purified water. Electrolytes are dissolved or suspended in solution, which create an electrical charge that is needed for the body to function. They help maintain stable blood pressure and circulation, regulate body temperature, transport nutrients, detoxify metabolic waste (heavy metals, toxic chemicals, etc.)

and lubricate musculoskeletal joints. Loss of fluids and electrolytes can occur as a result of physical exertion, prolonged exposure to the elements, an illness, disease, side effects of medication, or anything that causes symptoms such as excessive perspiration, respiration, urination, diarrhoea or vomiting. Athletes, senior citizens, individuals with an infection, cold, flu virus and those who work or play outdoors for extended periods may be prone to electrolyte losses.

Selectrolytes are available from Morin Laboratories, Inc.

Tel: (001) 877 856 4860
www.morinlabs.com

Similasan

Similasan strives to provide 'superior, proven, homeopathic and healthy formulas that are free of harsh chemicals without known side effects or drug interactions'. All Similasan products are homeopathic and, therefore, regulated by the FDA, unlike supplements or herbal products. According to homeopathic principles, Similasan products address the root cause of self-limiting ailments by stimulating the body to heal itself, thus returning the body to a state of optimum health.

Similasan products offer relief for the ears, eyes, sinuses and throat caused by allergies, hayfever or environmental conditions. I particularly recommend the Allergy Eye Relief.

Similasan products are available in numerous stores.

www.healthyrelief.com

Tissue Salts

Elizabeth Gibaud is a naturopath, dietician and author of *The Facial Analysis Diet*. Over the years I have referred many clients to Elizabeth, who need extra help concerning weight loss, modern-day maladies and skin problems. Her approach and training are unique, as is her record for achieving results. Elizabeth uses tissue salts as a main part of her prescriptive recommendations. The following are two brands of tissue salts we recommend. Both are available at many independent health shops and pharmacies.

Martin & Pleasance

For over 150 years Australian company Martin & Pleasance has provided an extensive range of natural remedies, including Schuessler Tissue Salts, based on a commitment to integrity, quality and innovation. They remain loyal to traditional preparation techniques that have proven their value and effectiveness over time. Martin & Pleasance is committed to using the best raw materials, the highest standard of facilities, and have the ultimate product trials.

New Era Tissue Salts

New Era Tissue Salt Remedies are homeopathically prepared in accordance with Dr Schuessler's principles. The mineral salts in soft, moulded tablets are present in highly assimilated form. The tablets are placed on the tongue, from where the minerals are quickly absorbed into the bloodstream. Homeopathically prepared tissue salt remedies are safe and it is not knowingly possible to take an overdose. New Era Tissue Salt Remedies are safe for children and for use during pregnancy.

Travel Guard

With international travel becoming easier and more affordable, exotic countries are increasingly popular as both holiday and business destinations. Travellers are now being exposed to novel foreign foods, standards of hygiene and water quality. Holiday food should be enjoyable, but digestive sensitivities can turn a great holiday into a misery. The answer is to ensure the best nutritional protection available. Taken daily, Travel Guard may help to maintain the normal balance of friendly gut bacteria as well as supporting intestinal health and well-being.

www.biocare.co.uk

Visualize

Made from herbal extracts, Visualize includes bilberry and lutein for strengthening the eye tissue. The eye drops help with inflammation, redness or discomfort due to stress, tiredness, allergies or contact lenses.

www.lifesmart.co.uk

Witch Doctor Gel

Witch Doctor Gel combines natural witch hazel extract with skin treating conditioners in a clear gel. Acts immediately to relieve irritation and itching, reduces swelling and redness and protects against infection. It can be bought at any chemist.

SPECIAL SUPPLEMENTS

Barlean's Organic Oils

The health benefits of flax are many and research studies have shown that as part of a healthy diet, high-quality flax helps to maintain many of the body's vital systems and functions. These include maintaining healthy cardiovascular and immune systems as well as aiding digestion and metabolism. Flaxseed is also widely recognized as promoting radiant skin, shiny,glossy hair and healthy strong nails.

A daily serving of Barlean's highest lignan flax oil gives you omega-3, 6 and 9 essential fatty acids as well as a generous helping of proteins, vitamins and both soluble and insoluble fibre. Barlean's oils are completely organic and from pesticide-free seeds, unlike the majority of competitor makes. Barlean's oils are unrefined, unfiltered, and protected from heat, light and oxygen. They are also guaranteed free of any GM foods.

Barlean's Essential Woman contains organic flaxseed oil, organic evening primrose oil, flaxseed particulate, isoflavones and saponins isolated from soy. It is an ideal balanced oil for women with pre-, peri- or post-menopausal complaints.

Barlean's Omega Man is for men of all ages who are striving to be their healthiest. Omega Man provides the ideal essential fatty acid and plant phytochemical formula to support optimal health. It combines the purest and freshest flaxseed oil, rare styrian pumpkin seed oil, lignans and phospholipid and phytosterol complex.

Barlean's is distributed by Healthy and Essential.

Tel: 08700 536 000
www.healthyandessential.com

BioCare

BioCare was founded by practitioners with many years experience in nutritional and biological science. BioCare has a diverse range of products including vitamins, minerals, herbals, plant enzymes, probiotics and specialized products that support the gastrointestinal tract. The entire range is suitable for individuals who are either allergic to or intolerant of standard manufacturing aids, and virtually every BioCare product is suitable for vegetarians and vegans.

In manufacturing, every effort is made to use the purest raw materials and to utilize organic ingredients wherever possible. Many raw materials are manufactured in-house. Encapsulation is preferred because it allows minimal use of excipients, and the Natrafill process – filling the capsules with nothing but the active ingredients – is also employed. BioCare offers products such as acidophilus (for balancing the gut), which is in pure powder form.

I always keep BioCare's Cranberry Plus in my medicine cabinet and take a bottle of it with me when I travel. It is the best natural cure for cystitis. Also, Biona Organic Pure Cranberry Juice is a wonderful addition to your diet that will help maintain a healthy urinary tract. With no added sugar, this juice is great on its own, mixed with other juices, added to yoghurts or as a tart topping with muesli.

BioCare products are available at most health food shops and pharmacies.

Tel: 0121 433 3727
www.biocare.co.uk

Candigest Plus

Anyone suffering from *candida albicans* should consider this product. Candigest Plus contains six key enzymes. Two of the enzymes digest the yeast organism cell wall. Three others digest the carbohydrates off which the candida feeds, thus starving it. The sixth enzyme – protease – is the secret weapon that no other anti-fungal product has. It can digest the protein nucleus of the candida organism to remove it entirely from the body. Clinical studies have shown that candida cannot become resistant to Candigest Plus so its effects are lasting.

Candigest Plus is available at health food shops.

Tel: 0870 774 7011
www.gutdoctor.co.uk

Immunecare Colostrum

Colostrum has 37 immune-boosting components and growth factors that help repair skin, bones, muscle and connective tissue to keep our bodies young. Colostrum is arguably nature's most effective immune-system booster. The 'first milk' produced by dairy cows in the days immediately after calving, it has a high concentration of proteins with antibodies. Colostrum is completely transferable to humans hence we can enjoy the significant health benefits including improved energy levels, increased concentration, assistance with pain control, promotion of healing and boosting of the immune system.

Immunecare Colostrum can be used to help a wide range of conditions. It can protect against colds, flu, ear, nose and chest infections. It helps heal wounds and minimize skin disorders. It minimizes the effects of autoimmune disorders including MS, lupus, scleroderma and rheumatoid arthritis. In addition, it can heal and protect against gastrointestinal disorders including IBS, colitis, coeliac disease, leaky gut and Crohn's disease.

It is available in the UK from Cornwall-based company Winning Team. Its founders, Neil Wootten and Janine Burns, discovered Immunecare Colostrum while travelling in New Zealand in 2000. At the time, Janine was suffering from ME and was advised by the dairy farmers there to take the supplement. It worked so well that she and Neil were determined to bring it to the UK so others could benefit.

It is available at health food shops.

Tel: 01752 203 018 (for supplies and personalized advice).
www.immunecare.co.uk

Medic Herb

Medic Herb products are high-quality, licensed herbal remedies. They contain standardized extracts of each herb and are supported by comprehensive clinical trials. By using scientific techniques to ensure the quality and effectiveness of each tablet, they have taken traditional natural remedies and brought them up to the standards of the modern world. Where possible, Medic Herb combines two or more herbs so that they work in synergy, maximizing their therapeutic effects to bring natural relief and restore harmony to the body.

Many of Medic Herb products are wheat-free, gluten-free, yeast-free, dairy-free, salt-free and GM-free. They are suitable for vegetarians and most suitable for vegans.

Tel: 01628 488487

www.medicherb.co.uk

MorEPA and MorDHA

Essential fatty acids play a vital role in supporting the health and regeneration of the cells. Without them we couldn't function. Omega-3 and omega-6 are the two essential fatty acids that we need. A reliance upon processed foods and those produced by modern farming methods has led to an imbalance in our diet: many of us receive 20 times more omega-6 than omega-3. The greatest concentration of omega-3 fatty acids are found in fatty fish and flaxseed oil.

Omega-3 taken from fatty fish contains what are known as EPA (Eicosapentaenoic Acid) and DHA (Docosahexaenoic Acid). It is the purity, potency and careful balance of the two that makes MorEPA and MorDHA so effective. Many fish oil capsules contain less valuable omega-3 and much more surplus fat. They may even contain contaminants such as dioxins and heavy metals.

MorEPA and MorDHA products are made exclusively from fresh deep-water fish, which are chilled down to −50°C to remove any impurities. MorEPA fish oil typically contains 78 per cent of valuable omega-3, has no trace of toxic elements, and you need only one capsule a day, compared to up to six of other brands. The optimum ratios help maintain the vital functions of the body throughout the different stages of life. MorEPA-minis and MorDHA-minis are available for children.

MorEPA and MorDHA are distributed by Healthy and Essential.

www.healthyandessential.com

Ocuvite Lutein

Researchers at Harvard have found that just 6 mg of purified lutein a day lowers the odds of macular degeneration (now the leading cause of blindness among those aged over 50 in the UK) by 43 per cent. But since our average intake of this vital eye-protecting nutrient is only a third of this amount (2 mg) there is a clear need for supplementation.

Just one daily capsule of Ocuvite Lutein provides a full 6 mg of free-form lutein (the only type of lutein naturally found in the retina), as well as safe levels of other eye protecting antioxidants vitamins C, E and zinc.

It is available from GCI Healthcare.

Tel: 0207 072 4267

Sage Organic

'As a small but innovative company, I applaud Sage for sticking to their principles to formulate a long overdue organic range of herbs, for the inspirational way they have combined nutrients and herbs for making supplementation less confusing for us all and for the way they went back to the lab to reformulate, strengthen and improve their range in accordance with their customers' wishes. They have excellent technical expertise and a dedicated behind-the-scenes team who understand the importance of integrity and making a real difference to the health and well-being of their customers.' Susan Clark, author of *The Sunday Times' What's The Alternative* column.

Sage Organic designed their dual-packs to help dispel the confusion over supplement taking by offering the consumer an all-in-one solution. As a result each dual-pack contains 30 capsules with organic herbs and botanicals in one section combined with safe levels of 30 multivitamins in the other. A perfect solution to food supplement taking and conveniently packaged to provide one month's supply. The five dual packs in the current Sage Organic range are Healthy Man, Healthy Woman, Pregnancy, Menopause and Vitality.

The Sage Organic Healthy Man dual-pack contains a minimum of 100 per cent of the Recommended Daily Allowances for 14 essential vitamins and minerals. These include zinc, vital for male reproductive health, and the antioxidants vitamins C and E, which help neutralize free radicals. Additionally, the herbal capsule provides organic ingredients including Siberian ginseng and gaurana to encourage a feeling of energy. Other nutrients include alpha lipoic acid, L-arginine and acetyl L-Carnitine to support male health.

The Sage Organic Healthy Woman dual-pack combines essential vitamins, minerals and herbs tailored to women's needs. Healthy Woman contains organic dandelion root, gingko biloba, burdock root, sage leaf and Siberian ginseng, along with the food supplements spirulina, acerola cherry and an organic vegetable blend. Flax seeds provide a source of omega-3 essential fatty acids and antioxidant support comes from grape seed extract. Healthy Woman also delivers a good supply of B-vitamins to help maintain healthy skin and the nervous system as well as antioxidant nutrients such as selenium, vitamin E and zinc, which help protect the body's tissues against free radical damage and can help to support a healthy immune system.

All Sage Organic products are certified by the Soil Association, approved by the Vegetarian Society and registered with the Vegan Society. They are free of GM ingredients, wheat, yeast, gluten, hydrogenated oils, processing chemicals, preservatives, colourings, salt and sweeteners. All ingredients are of non-animal origin and contain no animal derivatives.

Sage Organic products are available at Sainsbury's, Waitrose, Safeway's, selected Boots and health food stores.

Tel: 01672 811 777

www.sageorganic.com

Source of Life

Source of Life Liquid fuses essential vitamins, energy-packed phytonutrients and whole food concentrates into a convenient, all natural supplement, guaranteed to deliver a Burst of Energy®. This highly concentrated supplement includes Source-70 Whole Food Complex. This proprietary complex uniquely combines the comprehensive phytonutrient goodness of spirulina, alfalfa leaf juice and barley grass juice with soluble whole food concentrates that deliver more than 70 highly absorbable trace elements.

Source of Life is herbal based, hypoallergenic and vegetarian. It is free of yeast, wheat, corn, soy, milk, salt, sugar and starch.

It is available from Planet Organic and other health food shops.
www.naturesplus.com

Xylitol

Xylitol is a new sugar-substitute that is not only low-glycaemic, but helps to prevent tooth decay, which is why it is now being used as a sweetener in toothpastes and chewing gum.

Xylitol is a white crystalline sweetener that occurs naturally in berries, fruit, vegetables, mushrooms and birch trees. It even occurs naturally in our bodies, and has been shown to be completely non-toxic and safe to take (unlike many other sweeteners).

Recently, Xylitol has become very popular as a sugar substitute because it has been shown to dramatically reduce tooth decay and even reverse it when it is already present. It can do this because of its molecular structure which makes it unusable by the mouth bacteria that cause dental caries – plaque cannot grow with it. Also, as the saliva that contains Xylitol is alkaline, the calcium and phosphate salts in our saliva can start to naturally remineralize our tooth enamel in the places that they are lacking. This has a hardening effect on decay-softened enamel.

One of the added benefits of Xylitol is the fact that it is both a low-glycaemic sweetener and alkalizing to the body, making it an ideal sugar substitute for people on weight-loss diets and for those wanting optimum health without the 'sugar blues'. As it is low-glycaemic, it has become popular as a sweetener for diabetics.

Xylitol is available from The Really Healthy Company.
Tel: 0208 480 1000
www.healthy.co.uk

Note: Other quality supplements are provided by First Nutrition, Helias, Higher Nature and Solgar.

TRAVEL SUGGESTIONS

I recommend travelling with the following: Ainsworths' Travel Kit; BioCare Cranberry Plus; Citricidal; Lavera Sun Lotion; Natto NKCP (if applicable, for DVT); Selectrolytes and Travel Guard.

HOUSEHOLD PRODUCTS

Citrus Magic, Ecover and EcoLino

All the above manufacture an extensive range of products for everyday use in the home including washing-up liquid, multipurpose cleaner, toilet cleaner, washing powder, fabric softener, bathroom cleaner, air freshener and stain remover. Using natural, biodegradable, mostly plant-based ingredients these products provide a safe, effective alternative to the products currently in your kitchen.
www.citrusmagic.co.uk
www.ediblenature.com
www.ecolino.be

The Healthy House

The Healthy House was established in 1991 as a small family business. The Skelton family, through personal experience of allergies and chemical sensitivities, realized that there was very little information or products available to help people who suffer from allergies. The allergy market has changed in the last 13 years with more and more businesses plugging into this expanding need. The Healthy House remains one of the most well-informed and personally experienced allergy mail order businesses around.

The Healthy House provides products for allergies of all kinds including asthma, eczema, multiple chemical sensitivity, electromagnetic and geopathic stress, and seasonal affective disorder (SAD). Products include air purifiers, dust mite bedding, water filters, light boxes for SAD, as well as products for people suffering from skin conditions and solutions for hayfever sufferers.

With a large proportion of customers suffering from multiple chemical sensitivity, The Healthy House offers products to help combat and reduce the use of chemicals in our lives: laundry balls, non-toxic paint, cosmetics and cleaning products. The Healthy House also offers mattresses and carpets without harmful chemical fire retardants and pesticides in them, organic paints and a range of vacuum cleaners with the British Allergy Foundation Seal of Approval.
Tel: 01453 752 216
www.healthy-house.co.uk

Norstar Biomagnetics

Magnet Therapy is not a miracle cure, but it can provide a very safe, effective and non-invasive means of treating a variety of common ailments that are prevalent in our modern world. For anyone suffering from general stiffness in the mornings, lack of energy, chronic fatigue, arthritis, rheumatism or any form of bone degeneration, quality magnets can provide much-needed relief and healing, particularly by sleeping on a magnetic mattress pad and/or with a magnetic pillow.

The Magnetic Mattress Pad and Magnetic Pillow bathe you in deeply relaxing magnetic fields to help you get a better night's sleep. The body uses your sleeping hours to regroup – even bolstering your immune system – and a magnetic pad can play a large part in that restoration by easing you into a deeper, calmer and more restful night's sleep. Obviously, the more restful your sleep the healthier and more energetic you will be during the day.

Lilias Curtin, ART Practitioner and one of the first accredited Magnetic Therapists in the UK, provides the following guidelines for understanding and purchasing magnetic products.

When purchasing a magnet for your personal use, you should be aware of the following details, which should all be clearly displayed on the packaging:

•   How strong is the magnet? Look for two measurements: core strength and surface strength (core strength will be the larger number). Magnets of around 3,000 gauss in strength will have a deep penetrating effect.
•   Does the magnet have a north side and south side, or is it bipolar (i.e. a north and south field on the same side

of the magnet)? If the latter, be aware that one of these is normally dominant. Lilias recommends that you always choose a single pole magnet.

• Each side of the magnet should be clearly marked as to which is the north side and which is the south side.

• How long will the magnetic field last for? Good magnets should last 15–20 years. These will have a high neodymium content, which should be clearly marked on the packaging.

• The north and south sides of a magnet have two very different roles. The north side brings down trauma, swelling and bruising and will neutralize acidity in the body. The south will stimulate enzyme action, glandular action and growth, and will increase acidity in the body. Unless you are an accredited magnet therapist, it is not advisable to use the south side.

• If wearing a magnetic bracelet, wear it on the right wrist. Wearing it on the left can raise blood pressure.

• If you are using a magnetic product already, it is important to remove it from the body every four to five weeks for at least one week to avoid the body becoming over accustomed to it, thus decreasing its effectiveness.

• Magnets are phenomenal for helping with insomnia and many people use magnetic pillows and mattress pads to assist with this. The energy from the magnets calms down the circadian rhythm of the brainwaves, helping to induce a deep state of sleep. It can enable you to feel well-rested on only a few hours' sleep. Secondly, the magnets will encourage up to 300 per cent more blood flow and oxygen in an area. Magnetic energy penetrates every tissue, cell and muscle, meaning they all work more efficiently. Lastly, magnets will give the body the energy required to heal itself without depleting its own energy resources.

• Individuals with pacemakers, defibrillators or insulin-implanted pumps should avoid such products, as well as those in the first stages of pregnancy.

For expert advice on Magnet Therapy or to find an accredited Magnet Therapist, contact the British Complementary Medical Association.

For more information on Norstar Biomagnetics see: www.norstarbiomagnetics.com.

Respro

The Respro City™ anti-pollution mask offers a high standard of protection from the inhalation of primary pollutants associated with vehicle exhaust emissions. The City™ mask has a contoured design ensuring the mask seals comfortably and is manufactured from hypo-allergenic neoprene. This mask has been specifically developed to filter a wide variety of pollutants commonly found in major cities. With two essential Techno™ exhalation valves to allow unwanted heat, carbon dioxide and water vapour out it is an excellent way to protect yourself against urban pollution.

The mask filters out hydrocarbons , nitrogen oxide, sulphur dioxide, lead oxide, black smoke, pollen dust and building dust.

www.respro.com

Veggi Wash

Veggi Wash uses 100 per cent natural vegetable- and fruit-based ingredients to safely remove pesticides, chemicals, waxes and any remaining soil from fruits and vegetables before eating.

www.goodnessdirect.co.uk

CHILDREN'S PRODUCTS

Earth Friendly Baby

Earth Friendly Baby products are hypoallergenic and pH balanced to be gentle to your baby's delicate skin. Their products are also organic, environmentally safe and have never been tested on animals. They contain no artificial colouring, petroleum-based ingredients or any synthetic fragrance or detergents.

They are available at Green Baby and Plant Organic as well as other health food shops.

Green Baby

Started in 1999 by Jill Barker just after the birth of her first baby, Green Baby provides safe, natural, environmentally friendly products for baby, infant and mother including: childrenswear, baby basics, cloth nappies, toiletries and remedies, maternity wear, nursery and bedding, baby equipment and toys.

Green Baby supplies Tushies, the only gel-free disposable nappies available in the UK. If you cut open your current disposable nappies you can shake out white granules (acrylic acid polymer salts), which are used for absorbency. Tushies Nappies only use cotton and wood pulp for absorbency. Tushies also offer Unfragranced Wipes, which are produced using aloe vera and are hypoallergenic and alcohol-free.

www.greenbaby.co.uk

Nature's Plus Kids Greenz

Kids Greenz is packed with high energy, phytonutrient-rich green foods. Broccoli and spinach are nature's premier nutrient-rich vegetables, yet they are often the most difficult to get children to eat. Kid Greenz chewables are incredibly delicious, and each nutrient-dense chewable tablet is formulated with all natural tropical fruit flavours that kids will love.

Kids Greenz are available at Planet Organic and other health food shops.

DETOXIFICATION

Each of us has experienced the positive effects of detoxifying our bodies such as increased energy, mental clarity and feeling happier.

We all instinctively detoxify our bodies. Think about your average day: you are exposed to environmental toxins when commuting, at work you are in an air-tight building with numerous synthetic materials all around you, and either you or a colleague may smoke at lunch. It is likely that by the end of the day you are longing for a shower. Why? Cleansing and scrubbing our skin is one of the inherent ways that our body detoxifies. After the shower, you feel refreshed, more alert and more energized.

Detoxification may be the missing link to disease prevention, especially for immune-compromised diseases such as cancer, arthritis, diabetes, candida and fatigue syndromes. Our chemicalized-food diet, with too much animal protein, fat, caffeine and alcohol, radically alters our internal ecosystems. Even if your diet is good, a cleanse can restore the body's vitality against environmental toxins that pave the way for disease-bearing bacteria and viruses.

Industrial pollutants, pesticides, additives in our foods, heavy metals, anaesthetics, residues from drugs (prescription, over-the-counter and recreational), and environmental hormones are trapped within the human body in greater concentrations than ever before. Every system of the body is affected, from tissue damage to sensory deterioration. Many chemicals are so widespread that we are unaware of them. But they have worked their way into our bodies faster than they can be eliminated and are causing allergies and addictions. Almost everyone can benefit from a cleanse. It is one of the best ways to remain healthy in a destructive environment.

Our bodies detoxify naturally every day, eliminating or neutralizing toxins through the colon, liver, kidneys, lungs, lymph and skin. But in our world today body systems and organs that were once capable of cleaning out unwanted substances are now completely overloaded; thus many unwanted substances stay in our tissues. Our bodies try to protect us from harmful material by setting it aside, surrounding it with mucus or fat so it won't cause an imbalance or trigger an immune reaction. (Your body stores foreign substances in its fatty deposits – a significant reason to keep your body fat low. Some people carry up to 15 extra pounds of mucus that harbors this waste!)

To detox consider juice fasting, colonic irrigation, sweating (e.g. in a sauna) and herbal cleanses.

Aqua Detox
The Aqua Detox machine generates electromagnetic frequencies through water. When these frequencies come into contact with the approximately 4,000 pores on the feet, they produce a dialysis effect which expels toxins from the body's organs via the feet. The Aqua Detox has been scientifically proven to remove hazardous chemicals from the body including ammonia, nitrates, phosphates and heavy metals.

Aqua Detox can be used by people of all ages to combat the cumulative effect of numerous man-made, chemical and environmental toxins. The Aqua Detox has been proven to stimu-late all of the cells within the body. This allows the cells to release any build-up of toxins and regain their natural balance, thus enabling them to work more efficiently. As a result of the detoxification, recipients often experience more satisfying sleep, increased vitality and glowing skin.
www.aquadetoxuk.com or
www.liliascurtin.co.uk

Himalayan Sea Salt
See page 205 for more information.

Koyotakara
Koyotakara sachets contain processed wood, vinegar and natural resource extracts. You stick the sachets onto the soles of your feet before going to bed, where they activate more than 60 acupuncture points on the feet, absorbing toxins from the whole body. The soles of the feet are reflexive zones of our human organs and are where acupuncture points are centralized.

The colour of the sachets will change to grey or brown and will contain a lot of unpleasant, odorous fluid. This shows the toxins are being extracted, and the unwanted or unhealthy lymphatic fluid from the body has been absorbed through the soles. When used continuously, the colouration changes into lighter tones, which shows that the toxins in the body have been reduced.

Koyotakara relaxes muscles, activates body cells, enhances metabolism, improves the immune system, improves your sleep quality and makes you feel energetic.
www.koyotakara.com

Moor Mud
Moor Mud contains the essence of hundreds of herbs, plants, grasses and flowers as well as organic substances, vitamins, trace elements and minerals. Moor Mud is highly anti-inflammatory and researchers have found that it stimulates the body's natural production of cortisones. It is rich in fatty acids and fat-soluble substances that ease penetration through the skin. It is an ideal treatment for water retention and cellulite.

Nicknamed the 'skinny wrap' by spa staff, Moor Mud provides a truly unforgettable European spa experience. A superb treatment from head to toe, this ultra-rich, odourless mud promotes excellent therapy and relaxation. Over 1,000 plant extracts and trace elements are found in this natural mud which is applied and wrapped in warmth for 25 minutes.

The famous Austrian Moor Mud is one of the most effective natural products I have seen for the treatment of arthritis, chronic skin conditions and stomach ailments. It is also an excellent choice for a general detox programme. Extensive ailments can be treated with this amazing healing mud. Moor Mud is used to help ease joint problems, pain and muscle tension, arthritis and rheumatism. Moor Mud helps release stressful tension and has been clinically proven to balance hormones. (There is a two-year wait for this treatment in Austria – it's that good!)

Moor Mud has been used for decades in hospitals, clinics and spas all over Europe and is an accepted and effective healing treatment for many ailments, detoxification programs, anti-cellulite treatments and much more. The mud has potent, revitalizing properties that affect the entire system of the body. This has proven to be a very popular spa treatment product, leaving people feeling refreshed, toned and revitalized, with improved mobility and stability.
Tel: 0845 130 6768
www.moorhealth.co.uk

Shape Changers and the Detox Wrap
In June 2003, ITV's *This Morning* programme ran a piece on products which claimed they could improve the unsightly effects of cellulite. I was invited on the programme to talk about all the aspects that needed to be included when getting rid of cellulite. I met Deborah Rees, with whom I had an immediate connection, and as the managing director and creator of the company, Shape Changers, she had been invited to demonstrate their Detox Wrap Home Kit. The model used was a size 14 with noticeable cellulite on her thighs, which were wrapped live on air.

Before starting the wrapping process, both her thighs were measured and after only 45 minutes – normally an hour is recommended – she had lost two inches from each thigh and there was a dramatic visible reduction in her cellulite. Shape Changers were judged to be the best product of the six tested.

The Shape Changers kit, which contains a Natural Sea Clay formulation, works by entering the body through the pores to draw out the toxins which live in and around fat cells. The wrap itself acts like a giant poultice, drawing toxins out of the body. It continues to flush away additional toxins through the lymphatic system even after the treatment is complete.

The most popular misconception is that it is a water-loss treatment, therefore dehydrating and short-lived. However, this is not the case. The wraps are clay-based so they draw out the toxins held in and around the fat cells. Because it is not a water-loss wrap the results are measured in inches and not weight, so there is no need to worry about dramatic weight fluctuations that water wraps can sometimes cause. In fact, the more water you drink the better the results.

The ingredients of the clay are constantly being researched and then reformulated so that it will be 100 per cent organic and approved by the Vegan and Vegetarian Society. You also only use one tablespoon rather than a huge bag of clay so you are not left with a gritty residue.

Beware of unbranded salon wraps where you cannot check their claims and efficacy. Many salons just buy unbranded 'green gunge' from their local beauty wholesalers. For more information on the Detox Wrap Home Kit, visit:

www.shapechangers.co.uk

Tidman's Sea Salt for Bathing

Dissolved in a warm bath these sea salts will help to relax and soothe your body, bringing relief from muscular aches and pains. It is also considered to be an effective treatment for certain skin complaints and is recommended for post-operative and post-natal healing. Tidman's is a completely natural product, with no added perfume or colour and contains only the naturally occurring mineral salts left after the sun's evaporation of sea water. It can be found at all natural products and health food outlets.

THE IMPORTANCE OF WATER

Blue Water

Scientific research into the principle behind homeopathy has shown that water has a memory which is influenced by the things it comes into contact with. The human body, being 70 per cent water, depends on regular water intake for life. Johann Grander, award-winning Austrian naturalist and inventor, believes that the energetic quality of the water and its 'memory' can influence the body. He discovered a process to take Austrian mountain spring water and turn it into highly energized water. Many users of Blue Water have reported experiencing improved hydration, increased energy levels and improved skin conditions.

Blue Water is distributed in the UK by Ultimate Water Ltd.

Tel: 0208 400 9070

www.ultimatewater.co.uk

Lakeland Willow Spring Water

Since its launch in January 2003, Lakeland Willow Spring Water has become increasingly popular in the UK and Ireland as the UK's only natural aquaceutical. It was awarded the 'Best Designer Water' at the 2004 World Aqua Expo in Paris, confirming Lakeland's place as the primary aquaceutical water in the world. 'Willow', containing the ingredient trace salicin, has been hailed as 'nature's answer' to the growing demand for water that can deliver health and beauty benefits such as eliminating toxins and improving the look and condition of the skin.

Lakeland Willow Water was formed in 1999 but its real history dates back to the 12th-century monks of Cartmel Priory. It was they who discovered the unique taste of this remarkable water.

Lakeland Willow Water is the only bottled water on sale which contains trace salicin, which is derived from white willow bark. Today, it is extracted at source and bottled at a state-of-the-art, multi-million pound plant which is equipped with the most advanced facilities to ensure continuing quality and purity of the water.

www.lakelandwillowwater.com

Penta

Penta water is the fastest-growing bottled water in the US and is a leading product in health stores. In the UK it is now being adopted by a spectrum of users including therapists, practitioners, physiotherapists, chiropractors, doctors, nutritionists, dieticians, healers, trainers and spas.

Penta water is truly ground-breaking. Researchers have verified that Penta water is a unique, structured fluid. The US Patent Office recently granted Penta a patent covering not only the process but the composition of the water as well. Penta water uses high-energy soundwaves to restructure the molecules into small, stable clusters. These small clusters are able to more effectively enter cells, one molecule at a time, through channels in the cell membrane.

Researchers at the University of California proved that Penta water hydrates cells faster and more effectively than other waters. Researchers at Moscow University demonstrated that Penta improves the environment inside your cells – increasing intracellular alkalinity dramatically – increasing cell survival by up to 270 per cent. A study at the University of St Thomas, Minnesota, demonstrated a 15 per cent performance increase in endurance athletes.

With regular consumption of Penta water people report an increase in energy, an improvement in skin and hair condition, a better sense of well-being, enhanced weight-loss success and increased mental focus. It is also said to help combat jet lag.

Tel: 01635 551 277

www.teampenta.co.uk

Aquathin

Tel: 01784 221 188

www.pureh2o.co.uk

CONCLUSION

We and the world around us are constantly changing. No doubt in the time it takes for this book to reach your hands, yet more new ideas and regimes will have appeared in the fields of health, fitness and well-being. No book will ever provide all the answers, because no one philosophy or belief system is tailored to you personally. You, your body and advances in health are constantly evolving. The goal is to be able to adapt to the never ending changes throughout the different stages of your life. This book provides the guidelines for doing this successfully.

My vision was not to give you the ultimate cure, but to introduce you to different possibilities, to encourage you to consider (or reconsider) different options, and, above all, to understand how important it is for you to tackle your well-being from a multidimensional perspective.

So this is the end of my bit…and the beginning of yours. If up until now you have merely been reading this, and have not yet begun to explore the many options for improving your health, now is the time. No more excuses. This is a resource. Use it.

USEFUL ADDRESSES

Rosemarie Arroyo
Harvest Training
Tel: 0117 930 8888
info@harvesttraining.com

Lyndsey Booth
The Healthy Living Centre
282 St Paul's Rd
London N1 2LH
Tel: 020 7704 6900

Dr Shamim Daya
The Wholistic Medical Centre
57 Harley Street
London W1G 8QS
Tel: 020 7580 7537
www.wholisticmedical.co.uk

British Society for Integrated Medicine
The Regent Clinic
21 Devonshire Place
London W1G 6HZ
www.bsim.org.uk

Allen Carr
Tel: 0800 389 2115
www.allencarrseasyway.com
postmaster@allencarr.demon.co.uk
30% discount for anyone mentioning
Carole Caplin

Michael Garzon
83 Curtain Road, London EC2A 3BS
Tel: 020 7684 5565
www.mbt-uk.com
michael.garzon@mbt-uk.com

Michael Breen
MBNLP
Grosvenor Gardens House
35-37 Grosvenor Gardens
London SW1W 0BS
Tel: 0870 11 62657
www.mbnlp.com
info@mbnlp.com

British Psychological Society
www.bps.org.uk

British Association for Behavioural and
Cognitive Psychotherapies
www.babcp.org.uk

Paul McKenna
www.paulmckenna.com

Mike Duckett
Coaching for Success
Sheldon House, 3 Plomer Hill
High Wycombe, Bucks HP13 5JQ
Tel: 01494 473504
www.coachingforsuccess.co.uk
mike@coachingforsuccess.co.uk

Ron Bracey
Consultant Clinical Psychologist
Tel: 01243 774473
www.urbanpsychologist.com
info@urbanpsychologist.com

Jacqueline Flexney-Briscoe, Hon Sec
The London Physio Centre
STHPA
148 Harley Street
London W1G 7LG
Tel: 0800 085 0682
www.londonphysiocentre.co.uk
help@physiocentre.co.uk

Dr Marina Carew, BDSLDS, RCS
Lavender Barn Holistic Dental and Therapy
Clinic
Brewers End, Takeley
Essex CM22 6QJ
Tel: 01279 870077
www.greatsmile.org.uk
marina@greatsmile.org.uk

David Hefferon
The Ella Clinic, 12 Upper Wimpole Street
London W1G 6LW
Tel: 020 7935 5281
www.holisticdentistry.co.uk
david@holisticdentistry.co.uk

Triple O Dental Laboratories are able to put
patients in touch with dentists who carry
out functional jaw orthopaedics
info@tripleodentallabs.com

John Roberts
The Integrated Health Practice
Cote Royd House, 7 Halifax Rd
Edgerton, Huddersfield
West Yorks HD3 3AN
Tel: 01484 514451
www.integratedheealthpractice.com

Sarah Carolides, MA, MPhil (Cantab), Dip
ION
Nutritional Therapist
Results Health and Fitness Centre
Tel: 020 8540 1220
info@resultshealthandfitness.co.uk.
www.resultshealthandfitness.co.uk

Lilias Curtin, BCMA. Reg. MCMA
Full of Energy Ltd
92 Harwood Road, Fulham
London SW6 4QH
Tel: 020 7731 4715
www.liliascurtin.co.uk
Lilias@liliascurtin.co.uk

Bill Mitchell
ART-Dental Surgeon
26 Wilson Street, Largs
Ayrshire KA30 9AQ
Tel: 01475 672009

Huw Martin-Jones
Integrated Dental Care
1 Manor Place, Edinburgh EH3 7DH
Tel: 0131 225 9093
www.integrateddentalcare.co.uk
info@integrateddentalcare.co.uk

Tom Craig, MCSP SRP
Consulting Physiotherapist specialising in
energy medicine
Heathwood, 86 Hamilton Avenue,
Pollokshields, Glasgow G41 4HD
Tel: 0141 427 0756
energymedicine@tom86craig.fsnet.co.uk

Dr Evelien van Amerongen
Aspects of Health Centre for Integrated
Dentistry and Medicine
1a Falkners Close, Fleet
Hampshire GU51 2XF
Tel: 01252 614 818
www.address-stress.com
Aspectsofhealth@address-stress.com

Dr Ted Mortar
Bio-Energetic Synchronization Technique
(BEST)
Mortar HealthSystem
215 West Poplar
Rogers, Arkansas 72756, USA
Tel: (001) 800 874 1478
www.mortar.com

David Brown, Masseur
Tel: 07930 481031
db.therapy@virgin.net

Dr. Mary Hoptroff
Tel: 01792 869 209

Gutdoctor
Tel: 0870 774 7008
www.gutdoctor.co.uk

Barefoot Botanicals
Tel: 0870 220 2273
www.barefoot-botanicals.com

Dr David Harvey-Austin
30 Weymouth Street, London W1G 7BS
Tel: 020 767 2732
d.harvey-austin1@btconnect.com

Dr Rosy Daniel BSc MBBCh
Harley Street Clinic
Tel: 020 7299 9428

Health Creation in Bristol
Tel: 0117-949-3366

Institute of Heartmath
www.heartmath.org

Andrew Ferguson
Notting Hill Osteopathic Practice
Tel: 020 7937 2298

Fiona Collins and Marie Duckett
Aesthetics Ltd
30 Devonshire Street
London W1G 6PU
Tel: 020 7908 3773
fionamarie@ukonline.co.uk

Simona Arneodo
Maternity Consultant
Tel: 020 7497 3726
simonarneodo@aol.com

Dr Dietrich Konrad Klinghardt, MD, PhD
Klinghardt Academy For The Healing Arts
1 Upper Square
Lewis Road, Forest Row
East Sussex RH18 5ES
Tel: 01342 824007
www.klinghardtacademy.com

Institute of Neurobiology
P.O. Box 5023
Bellevue, WA 98008
Tel: +425-462-1777
www.neuraltherapy.com
aant@neuraltherapy.com

David Samson
Tel: 0800 634 0512
info@avantihypnotherapy.com
www.avantihypnotherapy.com

Dr Reinhard Voll
Alcoholics Anonymous
UK helpline: 0845 769 7555
www.alcoholics-anonymous.org

Al-Anon
AL-ANON Family Groups UK
Tel: 020 7403 0888
www.al-anon.alateen.org

Elizabeth Gibaud
152 Harley Street
London W1G 7L
Tel: 020 7486 3486

Keith Wilson
Albany Kickboxing
Tel: 0771 363 8233
kwilson_57@yahoo.com

Consuelo Fernandez Andia
Tel: 07967 312353
onefgtime@hotmail.com

The London Spine Clinic
Tel: 020 7616 7720
info@londonspineclinic.com

INDEX

ACKNOWLEDGEMENTS

I dedicate this book to my mother, Sylvia, who pioneered
the work that LifeSmart does today and whose unerring
strength, love and inspiration have kept me going.

And my thanks to the following:

My sister, Nicci, brother-in-law, Pete, and niece, Eloise, for your on-going
patience, nurturing and support.

Maria Herman, for being the backbone and phenomenal support and
organizer to me and everyone at LifeSmart.

Andrea Laurence, my friend and partner-in-crime, who ensures the
smooth running of LifeSmart, and, along with Joanna Yeftich, has
contributed many hours of research to this book.

The holiday gang of 2004, who restored my faith in humanity at large
and made me laugh again.

Holmes Place, for being a solid and consistent foundation throughout
the past trials and tribulations enabling me to keep my sanity by doing
what I love to do most – work.

My clients and friends who have been like soldiers around me,
protecting, encouraging, and never ever letting me forget what's real and
of true value.

Christena Appleyard and Sue Corrigan at Night & Day magazine, who
not only made it possible for me to have a voice in areas that matter to me,
but whose guidance and mentoring have been invaluable in helping me to
transfer my thoughts to the written word.

Lyndsey Booth, who has been as steady as a rock from the beginning
and is an exceptional and inspirational practitioner and speaker.

Sarah Carolides, for your dedication and expertise, Lilias Curtin,
Shamim Daya, Marina Carew, Jacqueline Flexney-Briscoe, Elizabeth
Gibaud, Andrew Ferguson, Ron Bracey and Dave Brown for believing in
what you do and for achieving honest results at the highest level.

Alka Johnson, for your vision and energy and honesty, for taking on me
and LifeSmart.

Anne West, Sue Croft, James Lakeland, Maria Grachvogel, Paddy and
Rebecca Campbell, Katie Thomas and Keith Bishop for your never-ending
support.

Barry and Debbie Clegg and Pauline Dower for their staying power and
patience.

Alan Samson and Lucinda McNeile, who have been incredibly
supportive and an integral part of this book.

Carole Green, Michael Dover, David Rowley, Clive Hayball, Austin
Taylor, Nigel Soper, Lucy Henson and everybody else at Weidenfeld &
Nicolson.

Ramsey Khoury and John Parnell and the rest of the team at Blumedia
for our logo and website, and for their tremedous and generous input.

Bharti Vyas where I go to get looked after.

All of the contributors and associations without whom genuinely this
book would not have been possible.

Adj and Niel for years of top-quality training and Rick Walsh for his
wisdom and standards from which those of us in the fitness industry have
benefited immensely.

Mike Christie for the 'The Body Politic'.

The charity Kidscan for giving me the opportunity to put something
back with integrity.

And, finally, in a world that is far from kind, I would like to thank certain
characters from the press, and others who will know who they are, for
making sure that I practised what I preached. And for reminding me that
what doesn't destroy you only makes you stronger.

First published in the United Kingdom in 2005 by
Weidenfeld & Nicolson
An imprint of The Orion Publishing Group
Wellington House
125 Strand
London WC2R OBB

Text copyright © Carole Caplin 2005
Design and layout © Weidenfeld & Nicolson 2005

Photography by Coneyl Jay

Additional photography:
Stefan Bajic: 136, 137, 138, 143, 153 (bottom), 157, 158 (top),
159 (top)
A C Cooper: 28
Courtesy of Dr Marina Carew: 67
Graham Jetson, courtesy of Lilias Curtin: 70, 72, 73
Alan Murray: 26
John Swannell: 2, 4, 168

Illustration by Tim Brown, courtesy HeartMath: 39

Make-up by Nicky Crancher
Hair by Paul Salltrick and Ross Taylor

A CIP catalogue record for this book is available from the
British Library

ISBN 0 297 84383 4

Designed by Clive Hayball and Austin Taylor

Printed and bound in Italy by Printers SRL and LEGO